UNDERGROUND CLINICAL VIGNETTES

PATHOPHYSIOLOGY VOL. II

Classic Clinical Cases
for USMLE Step 1 & 2 Review [103 cases, 1st ed]

VIKAS BHUSHAN, MD
University of California, San Francisco, Class of 1991
Series Editor, Diagnostic Radiologist

CHIRAG AMIN, MD
University of Miami, Class of 1996
Orlando Regional Medical Center, Resident in Orthopaedic Surgery

TAO LE, MD
University of California, San Francisco, Class of 1996
Yale-New Haven Hospital, Resident in Internal Medicine

HOANG NGUYEN
Northwestern University, Medical Scientist Training Program

JOSE M. FIERRO, MD
La Salle University, Mexico City
Brookdale University Hospital, New York, Intern in Medicine/Pediatrics

VISHAL PALL, MBBS
Government Medical College, Chandigarh, India, Class of 1996

ALEXANDER GRIMM
St. Louis University School of Medicine, Class of 1999

Cover Design: Ashley Pound

Editor: Andrea Fellows

This book was created with MS Word97 using the following typefaces: Garamond, Futura Medium, and Futura ExtraBold. The cases were developed in a master table and converted into pages by a macro written by Alex Grimm. The camera-ready copy was created on a Lexmark Optra R by Vikas Bhushan.

Printed in the USA

ISBN: 1-890061-13-1

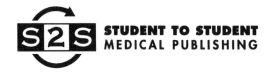

STUDENT TO STUDENT
MEDICAL PUBLISHING

Contributors

SAMIR MEHTA
Temple University, Class of 2000

VIPAL SONI
UCLA School of Medicine, Class of 1999

ALEA EUSEBIO
UCLA School of Medicine, Class of 2000

MARK TANAKA
UCSF School of Medicine, Class of 1999

Acknowledgments

Throughout the production of this book, we have had the support of many friends and colleagues. Special thanks to our administrative assistant, Gianni Le Nguyen. For expert computer support, Tarun Mathur (hardware) and Alex Grimm (software). For editing, proofreading, and assistance, thanks to Riva Rahl, Sundar Jayaraman, Carolyn Alexander, Warren Krackov, Julianne Brown, Arnold Chin, Sunit Das, Dr. Sonny Patel, Dr. Sana Khan, and Dr. Warren Levinson.

Table of Contents

Case	Subspecialty	Name
42	OB/Gyn	Inflammatory Carcinoma of the
43	OB/Gyn	Leiomyomata (Uterine Fibroids)
44	OB/Gyn	Leiomyosarcoma of the Uterus
45	OB/Gyn	Ovarian Carcinoma
46	OB/Gyn	Paget's Carcinoma of the Nipple
47	OB/Gyn	Papilloma of the Breast
48	OB/Gyn	Postpartum Thrombophlebitis
49	OB/Gyn	Preeclampsia
50	OB/Gyn	Vulvar Leukoplakia
51	OB/Gyn	Vulvar Malignant Melanoma
52	Pulmonary	Adult Respiratory Distress Syndrome
53	Pulmonary	Bronchial Asthma
54	Pulmonary	Chronic Bronchitis
55	Pulmonary	COPD
56	Pulmonary	Fat Embolism
57	Pulmonary	Lung Carcinoma
58	Pulmonary	Malignant Mesothelioma
59	Pulmonary	Pleural Effusion
60	Pulmonary	Pneumothorax (Spontaneous)
61	Pulmonary	Postoperative Atelectasis
62	Pulmonary	Primary Pulmonary Hypertension
63	Pulmonary	Pulmonary Embolism
64	Pulmonary	Silicosis
65	Pulmonary	Sudden Infant Death Syndrome
66	Pulmonary	Wegener's Granulomatosis
67	Pulmonology	Goodpasture's Syndrome
68	Rheumatology	Ankylosing Spondylitis
69	Rheumatology	Dermatomyositis
70	Rheumatology	Dupuytren's Contracture
71	Rheumatology	Hand–Schüller–Christian Disease
72	Rheumatology	Juvenile Rheumatoid Arthritis
73	Rheumatology	Mixed Connective Tissue Disorder
74	Rheumatology	Myotonic Dystrophy
75	Rheumatology	Paget's Disease of Bone
76	Rheumatology	Polyarteritis Nodosa
77	Rheumatology	Polymyositis /Dermatomyositis
78	Rheumatology	Progressive Systemic Sclerosis
79	Rheumatology	Reiter's Syndrome
80	Rheumatology	Rheumatoid Arthritis
81	Rheumatology	Sjögren's Syndrome
82	Rheumatology	Systemic Lupus Erythematosus (SLE)
83	Urology	Acute Tubular Necrosis (ATN)
84	Urology	Adult Polycystic Kidney Disease
85	Urology	Alport's Syndrome
86	Urology	Benign Prostatic Hypertrophy (BPH)
87	Urology	Diabetic Glomerulosclerosis

Case	Subspecialty	Name
88	Urology	IgA Nephropathy (Berger's Disease)
89	Urology	Membrano-proliferative
90	Urology	Membranous Glomerulonephritis
91	Urology	Minimal Change Disease
92	Urology	Nephrotic Syndrome
93	Urology	Papillary Carcinoma of the Bladder
94	Urology	Primary Amyloidosis
95	Urology	Prostate Carcinoma
96	Urology	Renal Cell Carcinoma
97	Urology	Renal Infarction
98	Urology	Renal Stones (Nephrolithiasis)
99	Urology	Renal Tubular Acidosis
100	Urology	Seminoma
101	Urology	Testicular Cancer
102	Urology	Testicular Torsion
103	Urology	Wilms' Tumor (Nephroblastoma)

Preface

This series was developed to address the increasing number of clinical vignette questions on the USMLE Step 1 and Step 2. It is designed to supplement and complement *First Aid for the USMLE Step 1* (Appleton & Lange).

Each book uses a series of approximately 100 **"supra-prototypical" cases as a way to condense testable facts and associations**. The clinical vignettes in this series are designed to incorporate as many testable facts as possible into a cohesive and memorable clinical picture. The vignettes represent composites drawn from general and specialty textbooks, reference books, thousands of USMLE style questions and the personal experience of the authors and reviewers.

Although each case tends to present all the signs, symptoms, and diagnostic findings for a particular illness, **patients generally will not present with such a "complete" picture either clinically or on the Step 1 exam**. Cases are not meant to simulate a potential real patient or an exam vignette. All the **boldfaced "buzzwords" are for learning purposes** and are not necessarily expected to be found in any one patient with the disease.

Definitions of selected important terms are placed within the vignettes in (= SMALL CAPS) in parentheses. Other parenthetical remarks often refer to the pathophysiology or mechanism of disease. The format should also help students learn to present cases succinctly during oral "bullet" presentations on clinical rotations. The cases are meant to be read as a condensed review, not as a primary reference.

The information provided in this book has been prepared with a great deal of thought and careful research. This book should not, however, be considered as your sole source of information. Corrections, suggestions and submissions of new cases are encouraged and will be acknowledged and incorporated in future editions (see How to Contribute).

How to Contribute

We invite your corrections and suggestions for the next edition of this book. **For the first submission of each factual correction or new vignette, you will receive a personal acknowledgment and a free copy of the revised book.**

We prefer that you submit corrections or suggestions via electronic mail to **vbhushan@aol.com**. Please include "Underground Vignettes" as the subject of your message.

For corrections to this book, visit our Student to Student Medical Publishing Site at:

http://www.s2smed.com

If you do not have access to e-mail, use the following mailing address: S2S Medical Publishing, 1015 Gayley Ave, Box 1113, Los Angeles, CA 90024 USA.

Abbreviations

ID/CC	identification and chief complaint
HPI	history of present illness
PE	physical exam

ABGs	arterial blood gases
CBC	complete blood count
ECG	electrocardiography
EMG	electromyography
LYTES	electrolytes
PBS	peripheral blood smear
PE	physical exam
PFTs	pulmonary function tests
UA	urinalysis
VS	vital signs

Angio	angiography
BE	barium enema
CT	computerized tomography
CXR	chest x-ray
Echo	echocardiography
EEG	electroencephalography
EGD	esophagogastroduodenoscopy
ERCP	endoscopic retrograde cholangiopancreatography
FNA	fine needle aspiration
HIDA	hepatoiminodiacetic acid [scan]
IVP	intravenous pyelography
KUB	kidneys/ureter/bladder
LP	lumbar puncture
Mammo	mammography
MR	magnetic resonance [imaging]
Nuc	nuclear medicine
PA	posteroanterior
PET	positron emission tomography
SBFT	small bowel follow through [barium study]
UGI	upper GI [barium study]
US	ultrasound
V/Q	ventilation perfusion
XR	x-ray

ID/CC A 9-year-old **white** female is brought to the ER by her parents because of breathing difficulty and productive cough with greenish sputum.

HPI The patient has a history of **recurrent upper respiratory tract infections** and **foul-smelling, diarrheic** stools **since infancy.** Overall, she has **failure to thrive.**

PE VS: tachycardia, tachypnea. PE: ecchymoses on upper limbs; hyperresonance to percussion with barrel-shaped chest; nasal polyps; scattered rales in both lung fields; hepatomegaly; clubbing.

Labs **High sodium and chloride** concentrations in **sweat test;** *Haemophilus influenzae* and *Staphylococcus aureus* in sputum culture. PFTs: increased ratio of residual volume to total lung capacity (RV/TLC). **Increased fecal fat** (= STEATORRHEA). ABGs: hypoxemia; hypercapnia.

Imaging CXR: hyperinflation; patchy atelectasis; **bronchiectasis.**

Gross Pathology **Mucous plugging** of canaliculi in pancreas and liver; thick, inspissated secretions blocking and collapsing alveolar spaces (= ATELECTASIS); saccular dilatation of bronchioles in lungs (= BRONCHIECTASIS); thick viscous plugs may cause **small bowel obstruction** in neonatal period (= MECONIUM ILEUS); pancreas small and cystic.

Micro Pathology Inflammation and hyperplasia of mucus-secreting cells; fibrosis and fatty change in parenchyma of pancreas with cyst formation; medial thickening of pulmonary arteries.

Treatment Antibiotics; diet management; aggressive pulmonary physical therapy and supportive measures; dornase (= PULMOZYME) via nebulizer; consider lung transplant.

Discussion **Autosomal-recessive** disease due to mutation in chromosome 7, with higher incidence in Caucasians; produces chloride and H_2O transport alterations in epithelial cells with mucous obstruction in **pancreas** and **lungs,** resulting in **pancreatic insufficiency** (steatorrhea) and *Pseudomonas* and staphylococcal infections in lung.

ID/CC A newborn boy is brought into the genetics department for a karyotype study.

HPI He was born of a **45-year-old mother** who feels that her child is **developmentally retarded** with **characteristic "mongoloid" facial features;** her pregnancy was uneventful.

PE Generalized **hypotonia;** flattened face and low-set ears; **macroglossia;** flattened nasal bridge and **epicanthal folds;** silver-white spots on the periphery of irises (= BRUSHFIELD SPOTS); single **transverse palmar crease** (= SIMIAN CREASE); left systolic flow murmur with widely split fixed S2 (due to an atrial septal defect).

Labs Karyotype: **47, XX; trisomy 21.**

Imaging KUB: **double bubble** (dilated stomach and proximal duodenum) due to **duodenal atresia.** XR-Plain: hypoplastic middle and terminal phalanges of fifth digits (= ACROMICRIA).

Gross Pathology Brachycephalic head; small brain with shallow sulci; hypoplasia of frontal sinuses; endocardial cushion defect.

Micro Pathology N/A

Treatment Surgery for congenital heart defects and duodenal atresia; training in specialized groups.

Discussion Most **common chromosomal disorder;** most frequently caused by trisomy 21 (due to nondisjunction); less commonly caused by mosaicism or a Robertsonian translocation; higher incidence as **maternal age** advances; higher incidence of cardiac defects, especially **endocardial cushion defects;** higher incidence of **acute lymphocytic leukemia** and **presenile dementia of Alzheimer's type.**

Kartagener's Syndrome

ID/CC   A 23-year-old male presents for an evaluation of **primary sterility** and a **chronic productive cough.**

HPI   He has had **recurrent sinusitis** and lower respiratory tract infections since childhood and occasionally experiences hemoptysis and dyspnea on exertion. He also has difficulty hearing.

PE   Malnourishment; clubbing of fingers; central trachea; bilateral basal crepitant rales and rhonchi in both lung fields; **cardiac apical impulse** visible and palpated **in right** (vs. left) **sixth intercostal space** (= DEXTROCARDIA); normal genitalia.

Labs   WBC/PBS: normocytic, normochromic anemia. Obstructive pattern on pulmonary function tests; **immotile spermatozoa** on semen analysis.

Imaging   CXR: heart apex directed toward right hemithorax; generalized cystic **bronchiectasis** with characteristic honeycomb appearance and "tram-track" lines.

Gross Pathology   **Saccular and fusiform bronchial dilatation** (= BRONCHIECTASIS); heart morphologically normal but located in right hemithorax.

Micro Pathology   **Absence of dynein arms** on electron microscopic examination of sperm and bronchial cilia diagnostic.

Treatment   No specific therapy available; antibiotics with postural drainage.

Discussion   Ultrastructural inherited (**autosomal-recessive**) abnormality in sperm tails and cilia of respiratory tract epithelial cells; characterized by absence of adenosine triphosphatase (ATPase)-containing dynein arms of outer microtubular doublets; leads to **nonfunctioning respiratory tract cilia** (frequent infections) and **immotile spermatozoa** (infertility).

4   Klinefelter's Syndrome

ID/CC   A 23-year-old white male goes to his family doctor for evaluation of **sterility**.

HPI   His history was unremarkable; the patient has been well all his life.

PE   Tall stature; **height greater than arm span and crown-pubis length greater than pubis–floor** (= EUNUCHOID BODY PROPORTIONS); scant pubic and axillary hair; **gynecomastia; testes** firm, **small,** and nontender to palpation.

Labs   Reduced plasma testosterone levels; **increased urinary gonadotropin** levels; **azoospermia** on semen analysis. Karyotype: **47, XXY**. Positive polymerase chain reaction (PCR) for X-inactive specific transcriptase (XIST) in peripheral blood leukocytes.

Imaging   N/A

Gross Pathology   Small, atrophic testes; gynecomastia.

Micro Pathology   Female sex **chromatin bodies** (= BARR BODIES) in cells; testicular fibrosis with hyalinization, atrophy, aspermatogenesis.

Treatment   Testosterone therapy for developing secondary sexual characteristics.

Discussion   One of the most common causes of male hypogonadism; due to excess of X chromosomes, usually one more (XXY); other problems include high incidence of breast cancer, chronic obstructive pulmonary disease (COPD), diabetes mellitus, and **mild mental retardation.**

ID/CC   A 7-year-old boy is brought to the optometrist to request a prescription for eyeglasses owing to **diminished visual acuity.**

HPI   The boy has an unusual **eunuchoid body habitus** with long arms and legs; a family history reveals similar body proportions in other family members. He is referred to his family doctor, who on careful questioning discloses that an **uncle** had **died** of a **ruptured aortic aneurysm.**

PE   Tall; **long extremities;** arm span greater than height (= DOLICHOSTENOMELIA); **long, slender fingers** (= ARACHNODACTYLY); **dislocation of lenses** (= ECTOPIA LENTIS); severe myopia; inguinal hernia; high-arched palate; flat feet (= PES PLANUS); **aortic diastolic murmur** (aortic insufficiency); funnel chest due to pectus excavatum; scoliosis of thoracic spine.

Labs   Increased urinary hydroxyproline.

Imaging   CXR/CT/MR: marked dilatation of ascending aorta. XR-Plain: thoracic and lumbar kyphoscoliosis. Echo: mitral valve prolapse.

Gross Pathology   N/A

Micro Pathology   Cystic medial necrosis of aorta may lead to **dissection, rupture, aneurysm,** or **aortic insufficiency;** elastic lung fibers tortuous and thickened; emphysema formation.

Treatment   Spine bracing; ophthalmologic correction; endocarditis prophylaxis; beta-adrenergic blockers; aortic valve replacement.

Discussion   **Autosomal-dominant** pattern of inheritance due to defective **chromosome 15 fibrillin gene,** a glycoprotein secreted by fibroblasts that is a scaffolding for deposition of elastin.

ID/CC	A 17-year-old white female presents with primary **amenorrhea** and **lack of breast development.**
HPI	She has a history of **low birth weight** and lymphedema.
PE	**Short stature; low-set ears; webbed neck;** cubitus valgus; low hairline; **shield-like chest with widely spaced nipples; harsh systolic murmur heard on back** (due to coarctation of aorta); hypoplastic nails; short fourth metacarpals; high-arched palate; **absence of pubic and axillary hair;** small clitoris and uterus; ovaries not palpable.
Labs	High serum and urine follicle-stimulating hormone (FSH) and luteinizing hormone (LH); **no Barr bodies** on buccal smear. Karyotype: **45, XO.**
Imaging	US-Pelvic: infantile streak ovaries. Echo: bicuspid aortic valve.
Gross Pathology	Ovaries look grossly fibrotic and atrophic.
Micro Pathology	Absence of follicles in ovaries; normal ovarian stroma replaced by **fibrous streaks.**
Treatment	Growth hormone and androgens for increase in stature; afterwards, estrogen.
Discussion	Most common karyotype is 45, XO; less commonly, mosaicism; frequent skeletal, renal (horseshoe kidney), and cardiovascular anomalies.

Acute Glaucoma (Angle Closure)

ID/CC A 5-year-old **Asian** female develops **sudden,** acute **pain** and **loss of vision** in the right eye after watching a series of family slides in a **dark room.**

HPI She had been complaining of seeing **"halos" around lights** at night.

PE Injection (due to vasodilation) of ciliary and conjunctival blood vessels; **hazy cornea;** loss of peripheral vision; **markedly elevated intraocular pressure;** shallow anterior chamber with peripheral iridocorneal contact by slit-lamp exam; pupils mid-dilated and unresponsive to light and accommodation; hyperemic and edematous optic nerve bed on funduscopic exam.

Labs N/A

Imaging N/A

Gross Pathology Pathologically narrow anterior chamber; eye hyperopic and **rock-hard** in consistency; synechia formation; Schlemm's canal may be blocked.

Micro Pathology Degeneration and fibrosis of trabeculae.

Treatment Analgesics, IV acetazolamide; topical beta blockers; steroids; pilocarpine; **laser iridotomy.**

Discussion Sudden increase in intraocular pressure; may be **precipitated by mydriatics** and upon leaving **dark environments** for well-lit areas.

ID/CC   A 49-year-old **male** immigrant who is a native of Guam has seen three doctors in his country and tried different therapies for marked, **progressive weakness** of his hands and arms together with **difficulty speaking,** wasting of both hands, and troublesome **fasciculations.**

HPI   He has no history of sensory symptoms, bladder or bowel dysfunction, fever, exanthem, dog bites, vaccinations, or spinal or cranial trauma.

PE   **Bilateral wasting of hands**; deep tendon reflexes absent in upper limbs; **muscle weakness;** positive Babinski's sign; stiffness and spasticity of upper limbs; **fasciculations;** normal fundus, sensory system, and cranial nerves.

Labs   LP: CSF normal. **Slightly elevated creatine kinase (CK);** normal thyroid-stimulating hormone (TSH), T3, and T4 levels; normal serum calcium and glucose. EMG: partial innervation with abnormal spontaneous activity in resting muscle and reduction in motor units under voluntary control.

Imaging   CT/MR-Brain: **brain normal.**

Gross Pathology   N/A

Micro Pathology   Nonspecific atrophy on muscle biopsy.

Treatment   Largely supportive; disease is progressive and fatal.

Discussion   Also known as **Lou Gehrig's disease;** characterized by slowly progressive, generalized motor muscle paralysis.

ID/CC	A 40-year-old male complains of the **"worst headache of his life"** and **double vision.**
HPI	He has been **projectile vomiting.** He has no history of fever or neck stiffness.
PE	**Papilledema on funduscopic exam; right eye deviated laterally and downward** (= RIGHT THIRD CRANIAL NERVE PALSY); other cranial nerves normal, no meningeal signs noted; motor system examination normal.
Labs	Routine laboratory tests normal.
Imaging	Angio-Cerebral: posterior communicating (PCOM) artery aneurysm. CT-Head: enhancing mass impinging over right third nerve.
Gross Pathology	N/A
Micro Pathology	N/A
Treatment	Endovascular or neurosurgical clipping of aneurysm.
Discussion	Congenital berry aneurysms are associated with **polycystic kidney disease** and **arteriovenous malformation;** they may rupture (during sexual activity, weight lifting, straining) and **cause subarachnoid hemorrhage.**

ID/CC
A 35-year-old woman known to have rheumatic mitral stenosis awakens in the morning to find the **right side of her body paralyzed.**

HPI
The patient also complains of **palpitations.** She has no history of fever, neck stiffness, vomiting, headache, or transient ischemic attacks (TIAs).

PE
VS: no fever; irregularly irregular pulse. PE: dense **right-sided hemiplegia; brisk reflexes on right side; right-sided Babinski present;** fundus normal; loud S1; apical mid-diastolic murmur and opening snap.

Labs
ECG: presence of atrial fibrillation confirmed in addition to P-mitrale. Blood culture sterile; routine lab tests normal; clotting time, bleeding time, and prothrombin time (PT) normal.

Imaging
Echo: left atrial thrombus. CT: scan performed after 24 hours reveals **infarct in posterior limb of left internal capsule.**

Gross Pathology
N/A

Micro Pathology
N/A

Treatment
Start heparin after follow-up; therapy guided with prothrombin time (PT); digoxin for management of atrial fibrillation; valvuloplasty or valve replacement after resolution of left atrial thrombus.

Discussion
Mitral stenosis with atrial fibrillation predisposes to thromboembolism.

ID/CC A 14-year-old white **male** comes into the emergency room because of **projectile vomiting** and a severe **headache.**

HPI He has a history of unexplained **short stature** and **polyuria.**

PE **Papilledema and optic disc swelling** (due to increased intracranial pressure) on funduscopic exam; confusion; visual field testing reveals **bitemporal hemianopia;** no other focal neurologic signs; no neurocutaneous markers or meningeal signs.

Labs N/A

Imaging XR-Skull: **enlarged sella turcica.** CT/MR: **enhancing, cystic, multilobulated suprasellar mass with ring calcification;** hydrocephalus (due to obstruction of foramen of Monro and aqueduct of Sylvius).

Gross Pathology Cystic mass with concentric areas of calcification.

Micro Pathology Mixture of squamous epithelial elements and delicate reticular stroma; gliosis seen at periphery; cholesterol-rich cystic fluid.

Treatment Surgical removal; radiotherapy.

Discussion Craniopharyngioma is most **common supratentorial brain tumor in children;** embryologically derived from Rathke's pouch remnants. It is a common cause of **growth retardation, diabetes insipidus** (compression of pituitary), **bitemporal hemianopia** (compression of optic chiasm), and **headache** (obstructive hydrocephalus). Bimodal age distribution; second peak in fifth decade.

ID/CC   A 62-year-old man is brought to his family doctor because of rapidly progressive **dementia** and excessive **somnolence.**

HPI   Five years ago, he received a **corneal transplant.** His wife states that she has seen a definite **change in** his **personality** over the past year.

PE   **Dementia; myoclonic fasciculations;** normal funduscopic exam; no other focal neurologic signs.

Labs   LP: **normal CSF profile.** EEG: bursts of high-voltage slow-wave activity and slow background.

Imaging   CT-Head: ventricular enlargement and cerebral atrophy. MR-Brain: increased signal intensity in affected areas. PET-Brain: areas of diminished glucose metabolism.

Gross Pathology   N/A

Micro Pathology   No inflammatory changes; amyloid deposition, **spongiform degeneration,** decrease in neurons of cerebral cortex, and astrocytic proliferation on brain biopsy.

Treatment   Usually fatal; vidarabine and amantadine are being tried.

Discussion   **Subacute spongiform encephalopathy** with very long incubation period; presumably caused by **slow virus or prion** and transmitted through corneal transplants, **dura matter allografts,** contaminated cadaveric growth hormone, or neurosurgical contamination. Lithium overdose may mimic signs and symptoms.

ID/CC   A 19-year-old female Olympic horseback rider is brought into the emergency room with **headache, confusion, weakness of the left side of her body, blurring of vision, and projectile vomiting.**

HPI   Three hours ago, she hit the right side of her head when she fell from a horse during a training exercise. She **lost consciousness** for one minute and then appeared to have **recovered completely** before presenting with the symptomatology (= LUCID INTERVAL).

PE   VS: BP mildly elevated; **bradycardia.** PS: **papilledema; **right-sided **mydriasis;** efferent pupillary reflex abnormality on right side; **deviation of right eyeball outward and downward** (= RIGHT CN III PALSY); left-sided weakness; brisk reflexes on left side; **extensor plantar response** on left side.

Labs   N/A

Imaging   CT/MR-Head: right temporal bone fracture; right-sided **lens-shaped** (convex) **hyperdense extra-axial fluid collection.**

Gross Pathology   **Collection of blood between dura mater and skull**, with mass effect.

Micro Pathology   N/A

Treatment   Emergent surgical evacuation.

Discussion   Results of arterial bleeding (rupture of **middle meningeal artery**) usually associated with skull fracture. Classically, patient loses consciousness immediately after head injury but regains consciousness and remains asymptomatic for variable time before symptoms worsen.

ID/CC   A 19-year-old male visits his orthopedist because of **ataxic gait,** congenital **clubfoot,** and **scoliosis** of the thoracic spine.

HPI   For the past several years, he has had **increasing difficulty walking;** the process began subtly, but he is now incapable of participating in sports. He also complains of a **progressive diminution of vision.**

PE   VS: **arrhythmia; tachycardia.** PS: bilateral concentric contraction of visual fields on visual field testing; findings suggestive of **retinitis pigmentosa** on retinal exam; scoliosis of thoracic spine; pes cavus deformity of right foot; diminished sensation in stocking-glove distribution; **proprioceptive sensory loss; areflexia; ataxia** of limbs; **Babinski's** sign; **forceful pulse; prominent jugular venous pressure; sustained apical impulse; S4** (due to hypertrophic cardiomyopathy).

Labs   ECG: left ventricular hypertrophy; inverted T waves.

Imaging   Echo: evidence of hypertrophic obstructive cardiomyopathy.

Gross Pathology   N/A

Micro Pathology   N/A

Treatment   No treatment available.

Discussion   Most common hereditary ataxia; **autosomal-recessive** disorder due to defective gene on chromosome 9.

ID/CC   A 60-year-old white male complains of **headache** that is worse in the morning along with occasional **nausea and vomiting** for six weeks.

HPI   One day prior to presentation, he had an isolated **grand mal seizure.**

PE   Bilateral papilledema; loss of recent memory; **brisk deep tendon reflexes** on right side; **Babinski** on right side.

Labs   N/A

Imaging   CT/MR: **irregular enhancing left mass** with **necrotic center; mass effect** and **surrounding edema.**

Gross Pathology   Hemorrhagic and necrotic tumor mass infiltrating left parietal lobe.

Micro Pathology   Biopsy reveals presence of anaplastic cells with pleomorphism and endothelial proliferation; **foci of necrosis** surrounded by palisading.

Treatment   Surgical resection; chemotherapy; radiotherapy.

Discussion   Astrocytomas are graded according to differentiation; **highest grade** (grade IV) **is glioblastoma multiforme.** Poor prognosis.

16   Guillain-Barré Syndrome

ID/CC   A 38-year-old male visits his family doctor complaining of **symmetric muscle weakness** that started **in the distal part of legs and has ascended gradually,** now involving the trunk and arms.

HPI   One week ago he suffered from **diarrhea and fever** and was diagnosed with and treated for *Campylobacter* **enteritis.**

PE   **Symmetrical** proximal muscle **weakness** and **flaccidity** in lower limbs; absent deep tendon reflexes; normal sensory exam; normal cranial nerves.

Labs   Elevated gamma globulin. LP: **increased CSF protein concentration without cellular increase;** normal glucose. Nonreactive VDRL; **decreased nerve conduction velocity** indicative of **demyelination** on electrophysiologic studies.

Imaging   N/A

Gross Pathology   N/A

Micro Pathology   N/A

Treatment   Plasmapheresis; intensive care and respiratory support.

Discussion   Common cause of **polyneuropathy** in adults; usually **preceded by** gastrointestinal or respiratory **infection** as well as by specific illnesses such as Epstein–Barr, *Campylobacter* enteritis, and cytomegalovirus infection; **respiratory paralysis** may occur, necessitating **mechanical ventilation.**

ID/CC   A **65-year-old** white **male** develops **sudden severe headache** and **right-sided hemiplegia.**

HPI   The patient is a **known hypertensive** and takes his medication irregularly; he is now **incontinent with regard to both feces and urine.**

PE   VS: **severe hypertension** (BP 210/180); no fever. PE: dense right sided **hemiplegia;** fundus exam reveals presence of **papilledema** in addition to **hypertensive retinopathy;** right-sided **Babinski;** eyes deviated toward left; no meningeal signs present.

Labs   Routine labs normal; LP not done, since intracranial pressure (ICP) raised.

Imaging   CT-Head: **focal hemorrhage** in left putamen region of basal ganglia.

Gross Pathology   Autopsy: mass of blood dissecting through parenchyma into deep structures of brain and ventricles.

Micro Pathology   Hypertensive changes seen in addition to putamenal hemorrhage; hyaline arteriolosclerosis; lipohyalinosis; Charcot–Bouchard aneurysms.

Treatment   Supportive management to **reduce intracranial pressure** and **blood pressure.**

Discussion   Bleeding is most often caused by hypertension. In the presence of moderate to severe hypertension, **small penetrating arterioles** may rupture deep within the brain, causing a **hematoma** that displaces brain structures. Common sites are the **putamen, thalamus, pons,** and **cerebellum.**

18 Medulloblastoma (with Obstructive Hydrocephalus)

ID/CC
A **6-year-old** male is brought to the emergency room with acute-onset **projectile vomiting,** severe headache, and blurring of vision.

HPI
The patient reports **unsteadiness of gait** that has progressively worsened over the past two months. He has no history of seizures, fever, or neck stiffness.

PE
Papilledema; no meningeal signs; nystagmus in all directions of gaze; truncal ataxia; cranial nerves normal.

Labs
CBC: slight anemia.

Imaging
CT/MR-Brain: homogeneously enhancing **mass in cerebellar vermis** compressing and filling fourth ventricle; **dilated third and lateral ventricles** (due to obstructive hydrocephalus).

Gross Pathology
Soft, well-circumscribed, light-grayish mass on cerebellar vermis.

Micro Pathology
Once intracranial pressure (ICP) controlled, CSF on lumbar puncture shows malignant cells; highly malignant tumor characterized by deeply staining nuclei with scant cytoplasm arranged in **pseudorosettes**.

Treatment
Corticosteroids for increased ICP; entire neuraxis irradiation; surgical extirpation; chemotherapy.

Discussion
Common tumor of **childhood;** most prevalent brain tumor in children less than seven years of age; classified as primitive neuroectodermal tumor (PNET).

ID/CC	A 59-year-old white female presents with a **severe, dull, retro-orbital headache,** vomiting, and **diplopia.**
HPI	She has **smoked** two packs of cigarettes a day for 22 years and has been diagnosed with **lung cancer.**
PE	VS: bradycardia; mild hypertension. PE: **papilledema** (increased intracranial pressure); **right oculomotor palsy** (right pupillary reflex abnormality in efferent pathway).
Labs	N/A
Imaging	CT/MR: round, discrete, **ring-enhancing lesion** in right frontal lobe; surrounding vasogenic edema; **shifting of midline structures to left** (> 1-cm shift considered severe).
Gross Pathology	N/A
Micro Pathology	Biopsy shows small cell carcinoma.
Treatment	Consider surgical resection; radiation therapy; dexamethasone (to control intracranial pressure).
Discussion	Blood-borne brain metastases commonly occur in patients with systemic malignancy. Common primary cancers that result in intracranial metastasis are lung, breast, gastrointestinal, and genitourinary cancer as well as melanoma.

ID/CC   A **36-year-old white** female pays an emergency visit to her ophthalmologist because of **loss of central vision and pain on movement of her left eye** (due to optic neuritis); she also presents with scanning speech and **intention tremor** in the hands.

HPI   Five years ago, she **emigrated** to the U.S. from **Sweden.** She has been suffering from **recurrent paresthesias in the hands, arms, and legs; weakness in the legs and arms; vertigo; bladder urgency** (multiple unrelated neurologic symptoms). Her family doctor told her she had "hysteria" and recommended psychotherapy.

PE   Diminished visual acuity; central scotoma found on visual field charting; **hyperemia and edema** of left **optic disk;** defective afferent pupillary reaction to light in left eye (= MARCUS GUNN PUPIL); **paresis of medial rectus muscle on lateral conjugate gaze but not on convergence** (= BILATERAL INTERNUCLEAR OPHTHALMOPLEGIA); **nystagmus** in abducting eye; electrical sensation running down back and into legs produced by neck flexion (= LHERMITTE'S SIGN); leg spasticity and increased deep tendon reflexes.

Labs   LP: **marked increase in CSF IgG concentration;** presence of **oligoclonal bands** in IgG region on CSF agarose electrophoresis; CSF otherwise normal. Abnormal visual, auditory, and somatosensory evoked responses.

Imaging   MR-Brain: multiple discrete high T2 signal abnormalities in **periventricular** and other white matter areas (especially **corpus callosum**).

Gross Pathology   Pathologic hallmark of disorder consists of distinctive small gray **plaques of demyelination** present in CNS white matter; optic neuritis.

Micro Pathology   Demyelination and gliosis; lipid-laden macrophages.

Treatment   Mainly supportive; corticosteroids; adrenocorticotropic hormone (ACTH); azathioprine; cyclophosphamide.

Discussion   Idiopathic demyelinating disorder; course marked by **intermittent remissions and exacerbations.**

ID/CC A 25-year-old **female** has had marked **weakness** and **drooping of the eyelids** (= PTOSIS) in the evening for the past four weeks; she does not experience any weakness in the morning following a good night's sleep.

HPI She has also been suffering from **double vision** (= DIPLOPIA) at the end of each day.

PE **Ptosis** develops on sustained elevation of eyelids; **dysphonia** develops as patient is asked to narrate complaints at length; **weakness of forward flexion of head develops after repetitive resistance to force;** patient could not maintain her upper limb in abducted position for more than a minute.

Labs **Clear-cut improvement in strength with edrophonium** administration. EMG: progressive decrement in voltage during repetitive, low-frequency stimulation of motor nerve. **Positive serum titer of antibodies to acetylcholine (ACh) receptors.**

Imaging N/A

Gross Pathology N/A

Micro Pathology N/A

Treatment Anticholinesterase (pyridostigmine); prednisone; thymectomy; plasmapheresis.

Discussion **Autoimmune disease** due to development of specific **antibodies to one or more ACh receptor subunits,** reducing availability of ACh receptors at neuromuscular junction. Thymoma present in 20% of cases.

ID/CC A 46-year-old white male complains to his internist of increasingly severe **headaches upon awakening** of a few months' duration; the headaches persist throughout the afternoon and are mild in the evenings.

HPI While in the doctor's office, the patient suffers a **seizure** and is brought to the emergency room.

PE Aside from mild papilledema, there are no significant findings.

Labs Normal.

Imaging CT/MR: large **frontal lobe mass** with focal **nodular calcifications.**

Gross Pathology Calcified cystic tumor with gelatinous consistency and areas of necrosis and hemorrhage.

Micro Pathology Tumor has **few anaplastic features;** regular cells aligned smoothly; spherical nuclei with finely granular chromatin, calcifications, and increased vascularity with areas of intratumoral bleeding.

Treatment Surgical resection/chemotherapy with radiation.

Discussion Usually low grade but may be anaplastic; oligodendrogliomas resemble astrocytomas in most respects but grow more slowly and are **more sensitive to chemotherapy;** calcification noted in 90% of cases.

ID/CC A 60-year-old male complains of **slow walking** and a **hand tremor** of a few months' duration.

HPI His wife also describes **postural instability, drooling of saliva, and generalized rigidity**.

PE "Mask-like" facies; mild involuntary pill-rolling tremor at rest; gait short-stepped and shuffling; "cog-wheel" rigidity; posture semiflexed; deep tendon reflexes normal; plantar responses bilaterally flexor.

Labs N/A

Imaging N/A

Gross Pathology Absence of brown/black pigment from **substantia nigra** (seen at autopsy).

Micro Pathology **Decreased pigmented neurons** in **substantia nigra** and **locus ceruleus;** residual neurons contain Lewy bodies, which are eosinophilic cytoplasmic inclusions with halos composed of dense aggregates of neurofilaments.

Treatment L-dopa; anti-cholinergics; amantadine; bromocriptine.

Discussion A degenerative disorder of the **basal ganglia** characterized by **rigidity, tremor, bradykinesia,** and **postural instability**.

Peripheral Neuropathy (Diabetic)

ID/CC A 40-year-old male with a history of **insulin-dependent diabetes mellitus (IDDM)** presents with **tingling, numbness, burning, and aching in the lower legs and feet.**

HPI The discomfort is particularly prominent at night and is often **relieved by walking.** A hoop over the feet to prevent contact with bedclothes is often helpful. The patient takes **insulin** irregularly.

PE Mild weakness; mild **distal sensory loss** and **loss of position and vibration sense** in both legs; bilaterally reduced ankle and knee jerks.

Labs Nerve conduction velocities slowed. EMG: features of **denervation.** Elevated glycosylated hemoglobin levels indicate poor blood sugar control.

Imaging N/A

Gross Pathology N/A

Micro Pathology N/A

Treatment Nonsteroidal anti-inflammatory drugs (NSAIDs) and carbamazepine effective in reducing discomfort; good glycemic control to slow progression of neuropathy.

Discussion N/A

ID/CC A 40-year-old male **dies** shortly after being brought to the emergency room with the **"most severe headache of his life."**

HPI His father died of chronic renal failure at the age of 45.

PE N/A

Labs N/A

Imaging CT-Head: **hyperdense blood** in cisterns and sulci.

Gross Pathology Brain reveals staining of inferior surfaces of brainstem, cerebellum, and cerebral hemispheres with fresh blood (consistent with subarachnoid hemorrhage, commonly due to congenital berry aneurysm rupture).

Micro Pathology N/A

Treatment N/A

Discussion In this case, hemorrhage was caused by ruptured intracranial aneurysm in patient with autosomal-dominant polycystic kidney disease. Other causes of subarachnoid hemorrhage include arteriovenous (AV) malformation and trauma.

ID/CC A 30-year-old black male complains of **constant bifrontal headache** and **blurred vision** of three weeks' duration.

HPI He has had mild intermittent **frontal headaches for the past eight months** and has become **irritable** and difficult to live with; for the past month he has been **extremely drowsy** and often sleeps for 30 hours at a time. Ten months ago, **he fell** from a moving vehicle and **lacerated his scalp.**

PE **Bilateral papilledema;** dilated left pupil; right spastic hemiparesis; deep tendon reflexes on right side are brisk; **right-sided Babinski; no meningeal signs** present.

Labs Unremarkable. LP contraindicated due to raised intracranial pressure (ICP).

Imaging CT-Head: **hyperdense crescentic extra-axial fluid collections (early); hypodense fluid collection with thick membranes (late).**

Gross Pathology Old blood encased in thick adherent brown membranes.

Micro Pathology Outer membrane composed of granulation and fibrous tissue with hemosiderin; inner membrane shows fibrous tissue only.

Treatment Surgical drainage of hematoma.

Discussion Traumatic lesion characterized by accumulation of blood between dura and arachnoid; caused by **laceration of bridging veins;** results in **displacement of brain** and possible **cerebral herniations.**

ID/CC   A 30-year-old man is referred to a neurologist because of progressive **anesthesia and weakness of both arms, occipital headaches,** and a **stiff gait.**

HPI   He has no history of significant trauma in the past.

PE   No motor deficits; **lack of pain and temperature sensation in hands and arms** (due to spinothalamic tract involvement), **but preserved position and tactile sensation;** unimpaired pain and temperature sensation below arms; dorsal columns uninvolved; proprioceptive sensation spared; **thenar muscles** of both hands **atrophied; areflexia in both upper limbs;** brisk deep tendon reflexes in both lower limbs.

Labs   Normal.

Imaging   MR/CT-Spine: **cystic dilating within central cervical cord.**

Gross Pathology   Spinal cord shows **central cavitation** in longitudinal and cleftlike fashion.

Micro Pathology   Hydromyelia is lined by ependymal tissue; syringomyelia is not.

Treatment   Surgical shunting.

Discussion   Syringomyelia may be primary (associated with Arnold–Chiari malformation) or acquired (post-traumatic, postinflammatory, tumor-associated).

ID/CC	An 18-year-old man presents with **headache, ataxia,** and progressive loss of vision.
HPI	His **father** died of metastatic **bilateral renal cell carcinoma** at a relatively **young** age.
PE	Cerebellar ataxia; **nystagmus;** past-pointing and **inability to perform rapid alternating movements** (= DYSDIADOCHOKINESIA); funduscopic exam reveals presence of **retinal hemangiomas** and moderate papilledema (due to increased intracranial pressure).
Labs	UA: normal (hematuria may signal renal cell carcinoma).
Imaging	CT/MR-Head: **cerebellar solid/cystic lesion** with **enhancing mural nodule.** CT-Abdomen: **renal, hepatic, and pancreatic cysts.**
Gross Pathology	**Hemangioblastomas** of cerebellum and retina; tumor occasionally located in medulla or cervical spinal cord.
Micro Pathology	N/A
Treatment	Surgical removal of tumor; photocoagulation for treatment of retinal lesions.
Discussion	Rare **autosomal-dominant** neurocutaneous dysplasia; gene has been linked to the raf-1 oncogene on chromosome 3; variable penetrance and delayed expression. **Associated with renal cell carcinoma** that is often multifocal or bilateral.

ID/CC   A 49-year-old male who is a known **chronic alcoholic** is brought to the emergency room with dehydration, jaundice, and fever; blood is drawn for routine tests and an infusion of **5% dextrose is begun, after which he becomes stuporous.**

HPI   He had been admitted to the ER several times before for alcoholic gastritis and acute intoxication.

PE   Patient **confused** and **stuporous;** normal fundus; **nystagmus;** skin and mucosal icterus; spider nevi on neck and upper chest; pitting pedal edema; abdominal distention with shifting dullness (= ASCITES); hepatosplenomegaly.

Labs   Increased serum bilirubin, predominantly direct; **low serum albumin; increased serum aspartate transaminase (AST) and alanine transaminase (ALT) (AST > ALT);** markedly elevated gamma-glutamyl transferase (GGT); mildly elevated alkaline phosphatase; slightly prolonged prothrombin time (PT); normal serum electrolytes and blood sugar; transudate revealed on ascitic fluid exam.

Imaging   US/CT-Abdomen: hepatomegaly and splenomegaly with evidence of free fluid in peritoneal cavity.

Gross Pathology   Micronodular cirrhosis and fatty change of the liver.

Micro Pathology   Neutrophilic infiltrate; "Mallory hyaline bodies"; piecemeal necrosis and fibrosis surrounding central vein of portal triad on liver biopsy.

Treatment   IV thiamine; complete abstinence from alcohol.

Discussion   Caused by thiamine deficiency (most common cause is alcoholism). **Alcoholics should receive thiamine before glucose** to prevent this.

ID/CC   A 22-year-old **female** presents with an **abnormal cervical Pap smear.**

HPI   She has no history of irregular menstrual bleeding, postcoital bleeding, intermenstrual bleeding, or vaginal discharge. She delivered her first baby at the age of 18 and has had **multiple sexual partners.**

PE   N/A

Labs   N/A

Imaging   Colposcopy reveals a suspicious area from which a biopsy is taken.

Gross Pathology   N/A

Micro Pathology   Loss of normal orientation of squamous cells on biopsy; atypical cells with wrinkled nuclei and perinuclear halos involving full thickness of squamous epithelium; basement membrane intact.

Treatment   Cone biopsy of area with regular follow-up examinations.

Discussion   Cervical dysplasia is a precursor of cervical squamous cell carcinoma; associated with **human papillomavirus (HPV) types 16, 18, 31 infection.**

ID/CC	A 29-year-old Vietnamese **female** visits her family doctor because of protracted **nausea, vaginal bleeding, dyspnea, and hemoptysis.**
HPI	Her history reveals one previous normal gestation and one spontaneous abortion as well as a dilatation and curettage four months ago for a **hydatidiform mole.**
PE	Vaginal examination with speculum reveals **bluish-red vascular tumor** and **enlarged uterus;** adnexa and ovaries normal.
Labs	**Markedly elevated** serum and urinary **human chorionic gonadotropin (hCG) levels.**
Imaging	CXR: **multiple metastatic nodules** (= "CANNONBALL" SECONDARY LESIONS).
Gross Pathology	N/A
Micro Pathology	Exaggerated trophoblastic (cytotrophoblastic and syncytiotrophoblastic) tissue proliferation with endometrial penetration; cellular atypia and hematogenous/lymphatic spread.
Treatment	Chemotherapy; follow-up with serial serum hCG levels.
Discussion	Malignant gestational tumor; may develop during normal pregnancy, after evacuation of hydatidiform mole, or after previous spontaneous abortions.

ID/CC A 45-year-old Hispanic female is brought to the gynecologist for an evaluation of a **gross difference in the size of her breasts** of recent origin.

HPI Her medical history is unremarkable. Despite the recent increase in the size of her right breast, she **does not feel any pain and feels only a sensation of fullness.**

PE **Very large mass** with **firm, "wooden-log" consistency** involving almost all of right breast, making it twice the size of opposite breast; **mobile mass;** appears **well circumscribed; collateral bluish veins seen on skin** along with striae; no peau d'orange appearance; no nipple retraction, axillary lymphadenopathy, or hepatomegaly; opposite breast normal.

Labs N/A

Imaging US: large, smooth multilobulated mass.

Gross Pathology Large tumor with numerous **cystic spaces on cut section of stroma, producing recesses and longitudinal openings** and causing a leaflike (phyllodes) appearance.

Micro Pathology Abundance of normal-looking ducts, acini, and stroma with no signs of cellular atypia and low mitotic index.

Treatment Simple excision.

Discussion Less common benign tumor of breast; also known as giant fibroadenoma. **Bulky tumor** that, although usually benign histologically, **may recur** following excision and sometimes undergoes malignant degeneration (5-10%). **Rarely metastasizes** to lymph nodes or distant sites.

ID/CC A 33-year-old Hispanic **multigravida** in her 20th week of pregnancy comes to the gynecologist's office complaining of a **mass in her abdomen.**

HPI She is **pregnant for the fifth time.** She has had no prior abortions or C-sections.

PE VS: normotension. PE: no edema; uterus correct height for gestational age (at level of umbilicus); **ill-defined, painless, nonmovable mass** 5 cm from midline on mesogastrium; skin not red or warm; no exudate; no fluctuation; **mass seems to disappear on contraction of rectus muscle.**

Labs Routine lab work on blood, urine, and stool normal.

Imaging CT/MR-Abdomen: circumscribed mass.

Gross Pathology Coarsely trabeculated tumor resembling scar tissue; appears to **arise from musculoaponeurotic wall.**

Micro Pathology Elongated, spindle-shaped cells; fibroblastic process; no evidence of atypical mitoses on biopsy.

Treatment Surgical excision; radiotherapy.

Discussion A type of fibromatosis of anterior abdominal wall in women; associated with previous trauma, multiple pregnancies, and Gardner's syndrome; **frequently recurs after excision.**

ID/CC	A 25-year-old **woman** presents with **amenorrhea** of six weeks' duration and **pelvic pain** over the past day.
HPI	She has a history of **vaginal spotting off and on** for the past two weeks and has been using an **IUD** for the past three years. She has no history of vaginal discharge and no urinary symptoms, and her previous menstrual history is normal. She has had multiple bouts of **pelvic inflammatory disease.**
PE	VS: normotension. PE: pallor; abdominal distention and decreased bowel sounds; **cervical motion tenderness;** uterus soft and slightly enlarged on pelvic exam; **soft, tender boggy mass in right adnexa and pouch of Douglas.**
Labs	CBC: anemia. **Human chorionic gonadotropin (hCG) levels lower than expected** for this period of gestation; culdocentesis reveals presence of blood in cul-de-sac.
Imaging	US-Pelvic: **no products of conception in uterine cavity;** doughnut-shaped mass in right adnexa; echogenic free fluid in cul-de-sac.
Gross Pathology	Extrauterine pregnancy, most commonly tubal.
Micro Pathology	Uterine curettage reveals presence of Arias–Stella reaction in the absence of villi.
Treatment	Laparoscopic linear salpingostomy and segmental resection; methotrexate.
Discussion	Other risk factors include **previous tubal surgery,** tubal ligation, **endometriosis, previous ectopic pregnancy,** and ovulation induction.

35   Endometrial Carcinoma

ID/CC   A 60-year-old **obese, nulliparous** white **female** presents with intermittent **postmenopausal vaginal bleeding** of three months' duration.

HPI   She has a history of **diabetes, hypertension,** and **infertility with polycystic ovaries; menopause began at 56 years of age.**

PE   **Uterus is not enlarged** on bimanual palpation; remainder of physical exam unremarkable.

Labs   CBC: mild anemia. Stool and urine tests within normal limits.

Imaging   US-Pelvic: **thickening** of **endometrial stripe.**

Gross Pathology   Hysteroscopic biopsy performed with dilatation and curettage; fungating mass visualized.

Micro Pathology   Adenocarcinoma.

Treatment   Radiation therapy; hysterectomy.

Discussion   **Estrogen-dependent** cancer; important differential diagnosis of postmenopausal bleeding.

ID/CC   A 27-year-old white female is admitted to the **infertility clinic** for evaluation of her **inability to conceive;** she also complains of **pain during intercourse** (= DYSPAREUNIA) and **pain during menses** (= DYSMENORRHEA).

HPI   She is **nulligravida.** On directed history she admits to having **rectal pain during menstruation;** she also complains of having an **abundant menstrual period** (= MENORRHAGIA OR HYPERMENORRHEA).

PE   **Bluish spots in posterior fornix** on vaginal speculum exam; **fixed, tender bilateral ovarian masses palpable** during menstruation on bimanual exam; **induration in pouch of Douglas** with **multiple small nodules** palpable through posterior fornix.

Labs   N/A

Imaging   Laparoscopy-Pelvis: ovaries adhere to broad ligament and show retraction and scarring in addition to **endometriomas,** with dense peritubal and periovarian **adhesions** and **thickening of uterosacral ligaments.** US-Pelvis: nonspecific cystic enlargement of ovaries.

Gross Pathology   Brownish nodules on uterosacral ligaments, ovaries, and pouch of Douglas.

Micro Pathology   Laparoscopic biopsy of affected areas shows nodules to consist of otherwise normal-looking, functioning endometrial glands.

Treatment   Oral contraceptives, progestogens, danazol, gonadotropin-releasing hormone (GnRH), surgical removal/coagulation of lesions.

Discussion   Endometriosis refers to endometrial tissue that is present outside uterus and that produces symptoms which vary with location. Endometrial implants (endometriomas or **"chocolate cysts"**) most frequently involve both **ovaries.**

Fat Necrosis of the Breast

ID/CC	A 27-year-old **woman** who is **actively training** for a marathon notes a **painful lump** in the upper outer quadrant of her right breast of two days' duration.
HPI	No history of fever; no known family history of breast cancer.
PE	**Retraction of overlying skin** in upper outer quadrant of right breast; **indurated lesion** the size of a lemon in same area; axillary lymph nodes not palpable.
Labs	N/A
Imaging	Mammo: **irregular mass** with **focal areas** of eggshell **calcification.**
Gross Pathology	Yellowish, fatty fluid on aspiration.
Micro Pathology	Excisional biopsy shows localized area of **granulation tissue** within which are numerous lipid-laden macrophages subjacent to necrotic fat cells.
Treatment	No other active management required.
Discussion	Unilateral localized process associated with **trauma,** breast biopsy, reduction mammoplasty, and radiation. Easily confused with cancer due to induration, fibrosis, dystrophic calcification, and retraction of overlying skin; key distinction is **presence of pain.**

ID/CC   A **25-year-old** black female visits her family doctor for a **painless** right **breast lump** that she discovered on self-examination; she is otherwise asymptomatic.

HPI   Her medical history is unremarkable.

PE   **Small, encapsulated, well-defined, rubbery, freely movable** 3-cm mass in right lower quadrant of right breast; no overlying skin changes; no nipple retraction; no lymphadenopathy; other breast normal.

Labs   All routine lab work normal.

Imaging   Mammo: oval low-density lesion with smooth margins; **"popcorn calcifications"** seen with degeneration.

Gross Pathology   Solid mass; no areas of necrosis or hemorrhage (central myxoid degeneration in older patients).

Micro Pathology   Glandular structures with ductal and stromal proliferation and no cellular atypia.

Treatment   Surgical excision.

Discussion   **Most common benign breast tumors in young women.** Sometimes enlarge during pregnancy or normal menstrual cycle.

39   Follicular Cyst of the Ovary

ID/CC   A 20-year-old Asian **female** visits her family doctor because of **chronic, intermittent left lower quadrant pain.**

HPI   The pain is not accompanied by dyspareunia, menstrual irregularity, vaginal discharge, abdominal distention, nausea, vomiting, or diarrhea. It is not correlated with her menstrual periods.

PE   **Left adnexal mass** on bimanual exam; uterosacral ligaments normal; pouch of Douglas normal; McBurney's point nontender; no evidence of ascites; remainder of exam normal.

Labs   Routine lab work on blood, urine, and stool normal; CA-125 levels not elevated.

Imaging   US-Pelvis: **large (5-cm) simple cyst in left ovary.**

Gross Pathology   N/A

Micro Pathology   Vaginal smears for cytohormonal evaluation reveal excessive estrogenic stimulation and lack of progestational effect.

Treatment   Follow-up by ultrasound (sizable percentage disappear spontaneously); laparoscopic removal if persistent.

Discussion   Most common cause of ovarian enlargement.

Hydatidiform Mole with Preeclampsia

ID/CC A 25-year-old Filipina in her **20th week of pregnancy** presents with **vaginal bleeding but no pain.**

HPI She has been feeling inordinately **nauseated** and has suffered from ringing in her ears.

PE VS: moderate hypertension (BP 150/95). **Uterus large for gestational age** (three finger breadths above umbilicus); lower extremity 2+ **nonpitting edema.**

Labs **Markedly increased beta human chorionic gonadotropin.** UA: **proteinuria** but no casts seen on microscopic exam. Elevated blood uric acid level. Karyotype: diploid XX (complete mole); triploid XXY or XXX (partial mole).

Imaging US-Pelvis: complex **"snowstorm" appearance** and **no fetal parts** in uterine cavity.

Gross Pathology Characteristic appearance of **clusters of grapes.**

Micro Pathology Chorionic villi markedly enlarged and hydropic with surrounding cyto- and syncytiotrophoblastic tissue proliferation and lack of adequate vascular supply.

Treatment Dilatation and curettage, periodic determination of human chorionic gonadotropin (hCG) levels to identify development of invasive mole or choriocarcinoma.

Discussion Gestational neoplasm; may present as painless vaginal bleeding, **preeclampsia** in first trimester, or **hyperemesis** gravidarum; may develop into **malignant choriocarcinoma** (20%).

ID/CC   A **52-year-old** unmarried white **nulliparous female** smoker with **early menarche** presents with a **painless lump** in her right breast.

HPI   The patient has a **history of atypical hyperplasia** of the right breast. Her **mother died of breast cancer** at 46 years of age.

PE   A 3-cm, **fixed, hard, and nontender mass** in **upper outer quadrant** of right breast; **retraction of overlying skin and nipple;** no nipple discharge; **palpable axillary lymph nodes** on right side.

Labs   Routine lab work normal; normal alkaline phosphatase (no bone metastases).

Imaging   Mammo: **spiculated mass with architectural distortion and multiple clustered pleomorphic microcalcifications;** skin thickening and retraction. CXR: no evidence of metastasis.

Gross Pathology   Hard, irregular whitish mass with granules of calcification and focal yellow areas of necrosis. Profound **fibrosis with induration** in stroma (= DESMOPLASTIC REACTION).

Micro Pathology   FNA: large pleomorphic cells arranged in glands, cords, nests, and sheets in dense fibrous stroma; tumor cells **estrogen and progesterone receptor negative** by flow cytometry. Core Biopsy: anaplastic cells with high mitotic index consistent with infiltrating ductal adenocarcinoma, not otherwise specified.

Treatment   Surgery; tamoxifen (for estrogen-receptor-positive tumors in premenopausal women); adjuvant chemotherapy with possible bone marrow transplantation; radiotherapy.

Discussion   **Most common type of breast cancer;** approximately 1 in 9 women in U.S. will develop breast cancer. Risk factors include **family history, early menarche, late menopause, obesity, exogenous estrogens, atypical hyperplasia of breast, and breast cancer in opposite breast.**

42   Inflammatory Carcinoma of the Breast

ID/CC   A 59-year-old white female comes to her family doctor because of a presumed "infection" in her right **breast;** she complains of **pain and swelling.**

HPI   Her history is unremarkable.

PE   VS: **no fever** or other systemic sign of infection. PE: right breast warm, **rock-hard, and swollen with no areas of fluctuation; one-third of breast erythematous** with shiny overlying skin having **peau d'orange** appearance; **painful** to touch and pressure; several axillary **lymph nodes enlarged and firm;** some **coalescent.**

Labs   Routine lab work normal.

Imaging   N/A

Gross Pathology   N/A

Micro Pathology   Large spheroidal cells and fine stroma infiltrated by lymphocytes on breast skin biopsy; lymphatic blood vessels occluded by tumor cells.

Treatment   Chemotherapy and radiotherapy, hormone therapy; poor prognosis.

Discussion   Breast cancer with angiolymphatic spread; malignant course with early and widespread metastases. Perform skin biopsy in patients diagnosed with breast infection who do not respond promptly to antibiotic treatment.

43 Leiomyomata (Uterine Fibroids)

ID/CC A 39-year-old **black female** presents with a several-month-long history of **profuse menstruation (=** HYPERMENORRHEA) **and frequent menstrual periods (=** POLYMENORRHEA).

HPI Further questioning also reveals **painful periods (=** DYSMENORRHEA) and increasing **urinary frequency**. She has a history of **infertility** and **recurrent spontaneous abortions.**

PE **Enlarged, irregular uterus** on bimanual palpation with several masses on posterior wall.

Labs CBC/PBS: hypochromic, microcytic anemia.

Imaging US-Pelvic: **multiple heterogeneous masses** distorting uterus.

Gross Pathology Occur in myometrium (95% are intramural) and are round, firm, and well circumscribed.

Micro Pathology Interlacing bundles of uniform, differentiated, elongated smooth muscle cells with few mitoses and no anaplasia; malignant transformation rare.

Treatment Myomectomy; hysterectomy.

Discussion **Most common tumor of uterus** and **most common tumor in women; estrogen-dependent.** Commonly occur after 30 years of age; tend to regress after menopause.

ID/CC   A 60-year-old woman visits her gynecologist because of a **foul-smelling, blood-tinged, purulent vaginal discharge.**

HPI   She has never been married and **has never been pregnant.** She is hypertensive and takes oral hypoglycemic agents for diabetes mellitus.

PE   VS: BP normal at present. PE: overweight; **fleshy, bulky, fungating tumor** protruding from cervical os on vaginal speculum exam.

Labs   N/A

Imaging   CT/MR: large, complex mass arising from uterus.

Gross Pathology   Large, fleshy tumor of myometrium with areas of necrosis and hemorrhage.

Micro Pathology   Background of spindle-shaped cells with **more than 10 mitoses per high-powered field** on biopsy; many mitoses have abnormal mitotic spindle.

Treatment   Adriamycin, progestins, combination chemotherapy.

Discussion   Very aggressive malignant tumor of myometrium; may arise in a leiomyoma or de novo; spreads by contiguity, hematogenously, and through lymphatics.

ID/CC	A **56-year-old white nulliparous woman** is referred for evaluation of a **pelvic mass** found on a routine physical.
HPI	She reports **increased frequency of micturition** and **irregular periods** until they ceased three years previously. **She has a history of breast cancer in the distant past.**
PE	**Large cystic mass** the size of a grapefruit in right pelvis that can be felt above the pubis symphysis.
Labs	**CA-125 levels elevated;** liver function tests normal.
Imaging	CT/US-Pelvis: **cystic pelvic mass arising out of right ovary.**
Gross Pathology	Partly solid and partly cystic mass.
Micro Pathology	Papillary structures of neoplastic ciliated columnar cells; **psammoma bodies.**
Treatment	Surgical staging and resection; chemotherapy.
Discussion	Third most common type of gynecologic cancer; **serous type** is **most common** and often bilateral. Often advanced at time of diagnosis (omental masses, liver masses, ascites).

Paget's Carcinoma of the Nipple

ID/CC   A 68-year-old white woman visits her dermatologist because of a longstanding **itching, painless, scaling, and oozing erythematous rash** over her right **nipple.**

HPI   Her **first menstrual period** started at **age 9,** and she has **never** been married or **had children;** her **menopause started at age 56.**

PE   **Nipple** on right breast **retracted** and appears **eczematous** with **redness,** some edema, and **desquamation; oozing** of yellowish exudate; painless left axillary **lymphadenopathy;** no hepatomegaly or lumps in opposite breast.

Labs   N/A

Imaging   N/A

Gross Pathology   Ductal carcinoma with extension to overlying skin.

Micro Pathology   Characteristic cells are mucin positive and have large nuclei and abundant, pale-staining cytoplasm (= PAGET'S CELLS).

Treatment   Modified radical mastectomy with axillary lymph node dissection and tamoxifen therapy.

Discussion   Scaly skin lesion in **areola and nipple** arising from **ductal adenocarcinoma** within subareolar excretory ducts and progressing outward.

ID/CC	A **35-year-old** female rushes to the emergency room and waits to see a doctor because she is concerned about a **bloody nipple discharge** that she discovered this morning.
HPI	She exercises, is very health conscious, and always has safe sex.
PE	Palpation around left nipple reveals **blood coming from one of the duct openings** and a **small, soft lump** beneath areola; no breast masses or axillary lymphadenopathy.
Labs	N/A
Imaging	Mammo: negative. Ductography: dilated duct with intraluminal filling defect.
Gross Pathology	Epithelial papillary growth with fibrotic components, characteristically located within a lactiferous duct.
Micro Pathology	No cellular atypia or anaplastic changes on specimen of bloody discharge; only blood intermixed with foamy macrophages and benign ductal epithelium with fibrovascular core.
Treatment	Surgical resection of lactiferous duct.
Discussion	Benign proliferation of ductal epithelial tissue. Most common cause of serous/sanguinous discharge.

ID/CC	A 28-year-old **woman** presents with **swelling of her entire left leg** of one day's duration.
HPI	She delivered a normal full-term male baby two days ago.
PE	Left leg **erythematous, warm, swollen,** and **tender.**
Labs	Routine tests normal; normal clotting profile.
Imaging	US-Doppler: clot in left femoral vein. Venography: confirmatory "gold standard" but usually not required.
Gross Pathology	N/A
Micro Pathology	N/A
Treatment	IV heparin and monitoring of clotting time and partial thromboplastin time (PTT); elevation of limb; analgesics and soaks.
Discussion	**Phlegmasia alba dolens** (painful white leg) is due to iliofemoral vein thrombosis occurring in late pregnancy and **post partum**; related to **compression by gravid uterus** and **hypercoagulability** of pregnancy.

ID/CC	A 30-year-old white **primigravida** at **36 weeks of gestation** visits her obstetrician for the first time in her pregnancy complaining of **swollen legs and headache.**
HPI	Her medical history is unremarkable, and her pregnancy has apparently developed with no complications until the onset of her symptoms.
PE	VS: **hypertension** (BP 170/110). PE: **excessive weight gain** (19 kg); funduscopic exam does not show changes of hypertensive retinopathy; 3+ **pitting pedal edema;** 1+ periorbital edema; fundal height appropriate; fetal parts palpable; fetal heart sounds normal.
Labs	CBC/PBS: complete blood counts and coagulation profile normal. Serum uric acid concentrations raised; lightly elevated aspartate transaminase (AST) and alanine transaminase (ALT); 3+ **proteinuria.**
Imaging	OB-US: single live fetus; lie longitudinal; presentation cephalic; normal biophysical profile; **placental infarctions** seen.
Gross Pathology	N/A
Micro Pathology	Endothelial cell swelling with obliteration of glomerular capillary lumen on renal biopsy.
Treatment	Antihypertensive agents; delivery of fetus and placenta, usually by C-section.
Discussion	Occurs in 5% of all pregnancies; most common during **last trimester of a first pregnancy;** characterized by triad of **hypertension, proteinuria, and edema.** Progression to eclampsia may occur, with visual disturbances, seizures, and coma.

ID/CC	A 75-year-old white **woman** visits her gynecologist for a routine checkup and is found to have **white spots** on her **genitalia.**
HPI	She complains of slight outer vaginal **itching** but denies any postmenopausal bleeding, vaginal discharge, or drug intake.
PE	**Hypochromic macules** on labia majora extending to perineum and inner thighs in patchy distribution with **scale formation** (= DESQUAMATION); **skin thickened and rough** (= HYPERKERATOTIC); no regional lymphadenopathy; atrophic vaginitis on vaginal speculum exam.
Labs	N/A
Imaging	N/A
Gross Pathology	N/A
Micro Pathology	Hyperkeratosis and fibrosis with thinning of squamous epithelium on biopsy; lymphocytic inflammatory infiltration, most prevalent surrounding blood vessels; no chronic inflammatory response; no signs of malignant transformation.
Treatment	**Biopsy**; subsequent treatment dependent on diagnosis.
Discussion	**Vulvar leukoplakia** is a clinical diagnosis that can be attributed to a variety of disorders that all produce white patches. Causes may be benign disorders such as vitiligo as well as inflammatory conditions, premalignant conditions (e.g., dystrophies), or squamous cell carcinoma. **Always perform a biopsy.**

51 Vulvar Malignant Melanoma

ID/CC A **73-year-old** woman is brought to a gynecologist by her daughter, who became aware of a **genital ulcer** while helping her mother shower.

HPI Her history reveals **weight loss** and **dyspnea** together with hypertension and arthritis.

PE Hard, nodular, 5-mm **pigmented and ulcerated** lesion on upper left **labia minora;** no inguinal lymphadenopathy; scattered crepitant rales on chest auscultation.

Labs CBC/PBS: slight anemia. Remainder of routine tests normal.

Imaging CXR: **multiple metastatic nodules..**

Gross Pathology N/A

Micro Pathology Lung biopsy reveals malignant melanoma cells with lymphocytic reaction infiltrating into underlying dermis; cells stain **positive for S100 antigen** and are **negative for mucin.**

Treatment Surgery with regional lymph node dissection and adjuvant chemotherapy.

Discussion Second most common vulvar malignancy (first is squamous cell carcinoma); metastasis and prognosis depend on extent of vertical growth.

ID/CC A 45-year-old white female is rushed to the OR because of **shock** due to postoperative bleeding; during intubation, she **vomits and aspirates** that day's breakfast.

HPI She had undergone a cholecystectomy two days before and had presented with postoperative bleeding requiring surgical exploration.

PE VS: **tachycardia; tachypnea; fever; hypotension.** PE: **central cyanosis;** warm, moist skin; **intercostal retraction; inspiratory crepitant rales** heard over both lung fields.

Labs CBC/PBS: marked **leukocytosis** with neutrophilia; fragmented red blood cells (RBCs); thrombocytopenia. ABGs: **severe hypoxemia with no improvement on 100% oxygen.** Increased blood urea nitrogen (BUN) and creatinine; increased aspartate transaminase (AST) and alanine transaminase (ALT).

Imaging CXR: typical **diffuse and symmetric parahilar ("bat-wing" pattern) alveolar filling** process suggestive of **noncardiogenic pulmonary edema.**

Gross Pathology Formation of **hyaline membranes** with proteinaceous deposits in alveoli; **pulmonary edema** with red, heavy lungs which, combined with **widespread atelectasis,** produces **stiff lung** with fibrosis.

Micro Pathology Endothelial and alveolocapillary damage with edema, hyaline membrane formation, and inflammatory infiltrate; **loss of surfactant** with fibroblast activity in later stages.

Treatment Mechanical ventilation, antibiotics, steroids, close monitoring of hemodynamic function.

Discussion Condition associated with **high mortality;** caused by gram-negative **sepsis, massive trauma,** burns, DIC, acute pancreatitis, narcotic overdose, and near-drowning. Characterized by diffuse alveolar capillary injury, which leads to increase in vascular permeability and pulmonary edema.

ID/CC   A 10-year-old girl is brought into the ER in **acute respiratory distress.**

HPI   The patient is known to be **allergic** to cats and pollen; her mother states that she had a **recent upper respiratory infection (URI).** She also complains of a history of moderate intermittent **dyspnea that is exacerbated by exercise.**

PE   VS: no fever; **tachypnea** (32); normal BP. PE: inspiratory and **expiratory wheezes** (due to bronchoconstriction, small airway inflammation); boggy and pale nasal mucosa; **accessory muscle** use during breathing; enlarged chest anteroposterior (AP) diameter; **hyperresonant** to percussion.

Labs   ABGs: primary respiratory alkalosis (hyperventilation). CBC: **eosinophilia** (13%). PFTs: Low FEV_1/FVC.

Imaging   CXR: hyperinflation with flattened diaphragms (increased residual volume due to **air trapping**); peribronchial cuffing.

Gross Pathology   **Hyperinflation** with air trapping in alveoli; **plugs of inspissated mucus;** edema of mucosal lining.

Micro Pathology   Inflammatory infiltrate of bronchial epithelium, mainly eosinophilic; plugging of airways with thickened mucus; hypertrophy of mucous glands; hyperplasia of smooth muscle of bronchi.

Treatment   Inhaled, oral, and parenteral bronchodilators; steroids; cromolyn; zafirlukast.

Discussion   Disease characterized by **hyperreactivity of the airways** and obstruction due to bronchospasm, edema, and mucus. Also known as **reactive airway disease.**

ID/CC	A 50-year-old white male **smoker** presents with **productive cough, copious sputum,** shortness of breath, and **fever.**
HPI	The patient has a **40-pack-year** smoking history. He has also experienced chronic dyspnea on exertion; chronic **productive cough,** usually **in the mornings,** for several years; and multiple colds each winter.
PE	VS: fever. PE: Stocky build with plethora; wheezes.
Labs	CBC: Elevated white blood cell (WBC) count (14,000); neutrophils predominant; **secondary polycythemia.** *Streptococcus pneumoniae* or *Haemophilus influenzae* on gram stain of sputum sample. ABGs: decreased PO_2, elevated PCO_2. PFTs: decreased vital capacity, **decreased FEV_1.**
Imaging	CXR: increased bronchovascular markings in lower lung fields.
Gross Pathology	Thick mucus secretion; edema of bronchial mucosa.
Micro Pathology	**Increased size and number of mucus glands** (Reid's index > 50); inflammation; fibrosis; squamous metaplasia.
Treatment	Antibiotics; bronchodilators; smoking cessation.
Discussion	N/A

ID/CC	A 58-year-old male presents with **chronic mucoid cough** and breathlessness of four years' duration.
HPI	He has an **80-pack-year smoking history.** He has no history of fever or chest pain but has had pedal edema for two weeks.
PE	Cyanosis; **pitting ankle edema; elevated jugular venous pressure; barrel-shaped chest** with bilateral rhonchi and fine inspiratory basal crepitant rales; **extended expiratory phase** breathing; no evidence of pleural effusion or ascites; mild tender hepatosplenomegaly.
Labs	ABGs: **hypoxia and hypercapnia.** CBC: **polycythemia.** PFTs: obstructive pattern (FEV_1/FVC ratio decreased).
Imaging	CXR-PA: **hyperinflation;** barrel chest; mild cardiomegaly; pruning of peripheral pulmonary arteries.
Gross Pathology	N/A
Micro Pathology	N/A
Treatment	**Cessation of smoking;** antibiotics; beta-2 agonists, corticosteroids; oxygen therapy and chest physiotherapy.
Discussion	Complications of COPD include right ventricular hypertrophy and right heart failure (= COR PULMONALE).

ID/CC   A 37-year-old **male** in the ICU develops **petechiae, altered sensorium, and marked dyspnea** that prove refractory to oxygen therapy.

HPI   **Twenty-four hours ago,** he was admitted to the hospital with **fractures of the shafts of both femurs, the pelvis, and the right humerus,** sustained following a fall from a 20-foot-high stepladder.

PE   VS: fever; marked dyspnea. PE: **delirium; central cyanosis;** using accessory muscles of respiration; wheezing heard over both lung fields.

Labs   ABGs: **profound arterial hypoxemia with hypercapnia.** CBC/PBS: thrombocytopenia. **Fat demonstrated in urine and sputum;** normal prothrombin and partial thromboplastin times (PT and PTT).

Imaging   CXR: early, normal; later, bilateral perihilar (= "BAT-WING") appearance of **pulmonary infiltrates** without cardiomegaly (due to noncardiogenic pulmonary edema). XR-Plain: long bone fractures.

Gross Pathology   N/A

Micro Pathology   Obstruction of pulmonary vessels by fat globules; chemical pneumonitis.

Treatment   Intermittent positive pressure ventilation with 100% oxygen, supportive management.

Discussion   Fat embolization usually occurs **24–72 hours after fractures of shafts of long bones.**

ID/CC A 58-year-old male presents with **breathlessness (=** DYSPNEA), **hoarseness, cough,** and **hemoptysis.**

HPI He has an **80-pack-year smoking history.** Over the past two months, he has also had a **significant loss of appetite and weight.**

PE Marked pallor; **cachexia; clubbing;** mild wheezing at rest; chest barrel shaped (emphysematous) and movements diminished on right; **dullness to percussion** over the right middle lobe; **no breath sounds** heard over right middle lobe, vocal fremitus reduced in same area.

Labs CBC: **normocytic, normochromic anemia.** Gram and ZN stains of sputum for acid-fast bacilli negative; sputum cytology reveals presence of **malignant squamous cells.**

Imaging CXR/CT: irregular hilar mass on right side, producing an obstruction atelectasis of right middle lobe. Bronchoscopy: right-sided hilar mass obstructing right middle bronchus.

Gross Pathology Postsurgical specimen reveals an irregular invasive mass of grayish-tan tumor spreading out from right middle bronchus and obstructing it.

Micro Pathology Biopsy reveals presence of malignant squamous cells, cellular stratification, **intercellular bridges,** and **"keratin pearls."**

Treatment Surgical resection can be potentially curative in patients with non-small-cell lung cancer.

Discussion Lung cancer is the **most preventable of cancers;** due to the increased incidence of smoking, lung cancer has exceeded breast cancer as the leading cause of cancer death in women. A **Pancoast's tumor** is a lung tumor located at lung apex in superior pulmonary sulcus that causes compression of cervical sympathetic plexus, resulting in **Horner's syndrome** (ptosis, miosis, anhidrosis) as well as scapular pain and ulnar nerve radiculopathy.

Malignant Mesothelioma

ID/CC A 67-year-old male is referred to a clinic for evaluation of **pleuritic pain, weight loss,** gradually progressive **dyspnea,** and a **nonproductive cough** of a few months' duration.

HPI He worked in a **shipyard** for 20 years before retiring, an occupation that involved **asbestos exposure.**

PE VS: normal. PS: **clubbing of fingers;** mild cyanosis; **reduced chest expansion;** end-inspiratory rales auscultated over both lung fields; **increase in vocal vibration transmission, dull percussion, reduced breath sounds, and egophony** in right side (due to pleural effusion).

Labs CBC/PBS: polycythemia; **marked eosinophilia.** PFTs: **restrictive pattern** observed (decreased vital capacity and decreased total lung capacity as well as increased FEV1/FVC ratio). Reduced diffusion capacity; pleural effusion bloody and shows acidic pH (< 7.3).

Imaging CXR: right-sided pleural effusion; diffuse bilateral **interstitial fibrosis; parietal pleural calcifications.** CT: highly irregular pleural-based masses; hemorrhagic effusion.

Gross Pathology Thick, **fibrous pleural plaques** with calcification; diffuse interstitial fibrosis; asbestos compounds form nest for further deposition of iron salts and glycoproteins (= FERRUGINOUS ASBESTOS BODIES).

Micro Pathology Epithelioid pattern of pleural malignant sarcomatous transformation with cellular atypia and high mitotic index.

Treatment Surgery; poor prognosis.

Discussion **Occupational exposure to asbestos** in 80% of cases, produces **lung fibrosis** with a **restrictive pattern;** asbestos and tobacco exposure synergistically increases risk of lung adenocarcinoma.

ID/CC A 37-year-old female comes to the emergency room complaining of **pleuritic pain** on the right side of her chest and **dyspnea** together with fever and a dry, nonproductive cough.

HPI There is no hemoptysis. Pain is typically **sharp and stabbing**, and it arises when she takes a deep breath (= PLEURISY).

PE **Decreased chest movement during inhalation** on right side; **dullness** on percussion of right lung base; **reduced or absent breath sounds** over right lung base; bronchial breath sounds auscultated on right side; friction rub; location of **dullness moves with respiration; decreased tactile fremitus** over right lung.

Labs CBC: elevated white blood cell (WBC) count with predominance of neutrophils. Gram-positive diplococci on sputum smear and culture; **elevated protein, decreased glucose, and many neutrophils in pleural exudate.**

Imaging CXR: consolidation of right lower lobe; pleural effusion on right side. XR-Lateral Decubitus: **layering of fluid** (therefore not loculated).

Gross Pathology N/A

Micro Pathology N/A

Treatment Antibiotics and needle drainage of effusion (= THORACENTESIS); sometimes obliteration of pleural space.

Discussion Effusions may be due to infection (viral, bacterial, mycobacterial, fungal); other causes are malignancies, congestive heart failure, cirrhosis, nephrotic syndrome, trauma, pancreatitis, collagen diseases and drug reactions. Effusions may be **transudative** (less than 3 g/dL of protein) or **exudative** (more than 3 g/dL of protein). Elevated pleural fluid lactate dehydrogenase (LDH) levels may be suggestive of malignancy. **Transudative pleural effusions** are commonly caused by CHF, cirrhosis, and nephrotic syndrome, whereas **exudative pleural effusions** are caused by TB, infections, malignancy, pancreatitis, pulmonary embolus, and chylothorax (milky pleural fluid).

ID/CC	A 25-year-old white **male** complains of **sudden pleuritic chest pain** and **shortness of breath** that **awakens him at night.**
HPI	He **smokes** one pack of cigarettes a day and states that his paternal **uncle once had a similar episode.**
PE	**Tall, thin** patient; diaphoretic and feels weak; left chest expands poorly on inspiration; trachea and apex beat displaced to right; left side **hyperresonant** to percussion; **decreased breath sounds; decreased tactile fremitus.**
Labs	ABGs: decreased PO_2; elevated PCO_2.
Imaging	CXR: partial collapse of left lung with no lung markings beyond **thin line parallel to chest wall; costophrenic sulcus abnormally radiolucent** (= "DEEP SULCUS" SIGN) in supine film.
Gross Pathology	Types: traumatic, spontaneous, tension, open; common causes: surgical puncture, rupture of emphysematous bullae, positive pressure mechanical ventilation, bronchopleural fistula.
Micro Pathology	N/A
Treatment	Pneumothorax evacuation via pleural catheter (= CHEST TUBE).
Discussion	Usual cause of spontaneous pneumothorax is rupture of **subpleural bleb.**

Postoperative Atelectasis

ID/CC A 50-year-old white male develops a **fever 24 hours after surgery.**

HPI He underwent an emergency **laparotomy** for a perforated peptic ulcer without any intraoperative or immediate postoperative complications.

PE VS: **fever;** normotension; **tachypnea; tachycardia.** PE: no cyanosis; **scattered rales** and **decreased breath sounds;** no calf tenderness; no hematoma, seroma, or discharge from wound; no inflammation of IV line veins; no urinary symptoms.

Labs ABGs: mild **hypoxemia.** CBC: slight neutrophilic leukocytosis. Blood and sputum culture sterile. ECG: sinus tachycardia.

Imaging CXR: **dense opacity in right lower lobe** (collapsed lobe) with elevation of right hemidiaphragm (due to volume loss).

Gross Pathology N/A

Micro Pathology N/A

Treatment Chest physiotherapy (incentive spirometry); deep inspirations; mucolytic agents.

Discussion Most common cause of postoperative fever in first 48 hours; alveolar collapse produced by occlusion due to viscid secretions favored by recumbency, hypoventilation, and oversedation. Other causes of postoperative fever, usually seen later in postoperative period, include urinary tract infection, IV catheter infection, deep venous thrombosis, wound infection, and drug reactions.

ID/CC	A **34-year-old** white obese **female** complains of **shortness of breath,** dizziness, and near-fainting spells.
HPI	She has been taking **prescription medication** for approximately six months in order to **lose weight.**
PE	Obesity; mild cyanosis; **large "a" wave** in jugular venous pressure; left parasternal heave; **loud S2;** narrow splitting of S2; rales on both bases; hepatomegaly.
Labs	CBC: **polycythemia.** ECG: **right axis deviation; right ventricle and right atrial hypertrophy.** ABGs: hypoxemia.
Imaging	CXR: enlarged right ventricle; enlarged main pulmonary artery with peripheral pruning.
Gross Pathology	Enlarged right ventricle with myocardial fiber hypertrophy; atherosclerosis of pulmonary artery; narrowing of arterioles.
Micro Pathology	Foci of hemorrhages in pulmonary parenchyma; hypertrophy of pulmonary vascular muscle; fibrosis; hemosiderin-laden macrophages (= "HEART FAILURE" CELLS).
Treatment	Calcium channel blockers; prostacyclin; inhaled nitric oxide; phlebotomy; heart-lung transplantation can be considered.
Discussion	Pathologic increase in pulmonary artery pressure; if longstanding, causes fatal right heart failure; may be primary (idiopathic) or secondary to intrinsic pulmonary disease.

ID/CC   A 60-year-old female who had undergone right **total hip replacement** presents on the sixth postoperative day with central **chest pain** and **acute-onset dyspnea.**

HPI   She has been immobile since the surgery.

PE   VS: low-grade fever; tachycardia; **tachypnea; hypotension.** PE: central cyanosis; **elevated jugular venous pressure; right ventricular gallop rhythm with widely split S2.**

Labs   ABGs: **hypoxia and hypercapnia** (type 2 respiratory failure). ECG: **S1Q3T3** pattern and sinus **tachycardia.**

Imaging   US-Doppler: **clot in right common femoral** vein. CXR: right lower lobe atelectasis. V/Q: three areas of ventilation-perfusion mismatch in right lung. Angio-Pulmonary: confirmatory; not required if V/Q scan is high probability.

Gross Pathology   Large thrombus seen in pulmonary artery.

Micro Pathology   Large occlusive thrombus seen in pulmonary artery with variable degree of recanalization.

Treatment   Supportive; thrombolytic therapy; consider embolectomy; heparin, Coumadin, and low molecular weight heparin (enoxaparin) instituted for prophylaxis (monitor INR).

Discussion   Pulmonary emboli most commonly originate from proximal deep venous thrombosis. Pulmonary angiography is gold standard in diagnosis of pulmonary embolism, but obtain a V/Q scan initially if clinically suspected. **Virchow's triad,** which outlines the risk factors of thrombus formation, includes blood stasis (e.g., immobilization), endothelial damage (e.g., surgery), and hypercoagulable states (e.g., malignancy, pregnancy, severe burns). Large emboli may cause cardiovascular collapse and sudden death.

ID/CC	A 56-year-old male presents with progressively increasing **dyspnea** and **dry cough** of several years' duration.
HPI	He is a nonsmoker, but his occupational history includes **mining and quarrying.**
PE	No clubbing, cyanosis, or lymphadenopathy; **reduced chest expansion** on inspiration; **dry inspiratory crackles** auscultated in upper lobes of both lungs.
Labs	PFTs: combined **obstructive and restrictive pattern** of functional impairment. Bronchoscopically guided lung biopsy establishes diagnosis; negative Mantoux test; sputum cytology and staining for acid-fast bacilli negative
Imaging	CXR-PA: rounded small opacities in upper lobes with retraction and **hilar lymphadenopathy; "eggshell" calcification of lymph nodes.**
Gross Pathology	Dense, small collagenous nodules in the upper lungs in the early stages; spread and become more diffuse as disease progresses.
Micro Pathology	Hyalinized whorls of collagen with little or no inflammation; polarized light demonstrates silica particles within nodules.
Treatment	Supportive; avoidance of further exposure.
Discussion	There is **increased incidence of tuberculosis** in silicosis patients. Silicosis leads to restrictive lung disease that varies in severity from mild to disabling.

65   Sudden Infant Death Syndrome (SIDS)

ID/CC   Paramedics are called at 7:00 a.m. because a **2-month-old male,** the child of Cuban immigrants, cannot be awakened by his mother; upon arrival, it is clear that the child has been dead for at least four hours.

HPI   The child was slightly premature, but aside from this, his history was unremarkable. There was nothing that could directly explain the episode. On directed history, **the mother admits to being a smoker and remembers that the child had had an upper respiratory infection four days ago.**

PE   No pathologic cause revealed that could explain death.

Labs   N/A

Imaging   N/A

Gross Pathology   Autopsy: petechiae on pleural and pericardial surfaces, pulmonary congestion, and scattered foci of lymphocytic tissue in interstitium of lungs.

Micro Pathology   N/A

Treatment   N/A

Discussion   SIDS refers to **death of an infant under one year** of age, usually during sleep, in which **death remains unexplained** even after complete autopsy; most have history of minor upper respiratory infection.

ID/CC   A 45-year-old white **male** complains of chronic nasal congestion and discharge over the past five months.

HPI   Ten days ago he developed an earache and cough together with bloody sputum production, dyspnea, muscle pain, red eyes, fever, and night sweats.

PE   Dried-up crusts of mucus in congestive nasal mucosa with shallow **ulcers and perforation of the nasal septum;** sibilant rales disseminated in lung fields.

Labs   CBC: mild anemia; moderate leukocytosis. UA: numerous red blood cells (RBCs); **red cell casts** and granular casts in urine. **Positive C-ANCA** in serum.

Imaging   CXR: scattered small nodular densities bilaterally with no hilar adenopathy (vs. sarcoid).

Gross Pathology   Granuloma formation in lungs; vasculitis and inflammation involving upper **respiratory tract,** lungs, peripheral arteries, and **kidneys.**

Micro Pathology   Focal necrotizing vasculitis involving small vessels; granulomas and crescentic glomerulonephritis.

Treatment   Immunosuppressive therapy with steroids and cyclophosphamide.

Discussion   Wegener's granulomatosis is a systemic autoimmune vasculitis that consists of necrotizing vasculitis and necrotizing granulomas of the lungs and airways, as well as necrotizing glomerulitis. Cytoplasmic antineutrophilic antibodies (C-ANCA) are seen in large majority of patients and serve as marker of disease activity.

Goodpasture's Syndrome

ID/CC   A **36-year-old** white **male** complains of a chronic cough of several months' duration, accompanied by lightheadedness, fatigue, and malaise; yesterday he **coughed up blood.**

HPI   He also describes intermittent fever and headaches in addition to small volumes of **dark orange urine.** He denies alcohol use but admits to being a heavy **smoker.**

PE   Diffuse pulmonary crackles bilaterally.

Labs   Azotemia. UA: oliguria; **hematuria;** proteinuria. **Iron deficiency anemia;** blood detected in sputum. ABGs: hypoxemia.

Imaging   CXR: bilateral alveolar infiltrates.

Gross Pathology   Increase in weight of **lungs** with areas of necrosis; **kidneys** enlarged and pale with decreased consistency.

Micro Pathology   Proliferative, necrotizing, crescentic **glomerulonephritis** on kidney biopsy with accumulation of neutrophils and macrophages in Bowman's capsule; characteristic **linear IgG deposits in glomerular basement membrane and alveolar septa** on immunofluorescence; anti-glomerular basement membrane protein in serum; necrotizing hemorrhagic **alveolitis** on lung biopsy.

Treatment   Plasma exchange; corticosteroids; immunosuppressive therapy.

Discussion   Hemorrhagic alveolitis with nephritis and iron deficiency anemia caused by anti-glomerular basement membrane antibodies (type II hypersensitivity reaction).

ID/CC A 24-year-old **white male** visits his family doctor complaining of **low-back pain and stiffness** on active movement of the spine for almost one year, increasing in severity.

HPI The pain increases with movement and radiates down the posterior thigh, improving as the day progresses.

PE **Stooped posture;** loss of lumbar lordosis and **fixed kyphosis; tenderness over sacroiliac joints;** reduced chest expansion; prominent abdomen.

Labs Elevated erythrocyte sedimentation rate (ESR); **negative rheumatoid tests; positive HLA-B27.**

Imaging XR-Plain: sclerosis and blurring of margins of **sacroiliac joints; ankylosis and fusion of vertebrae** (= "BAMBOO SPINE") in longstanding cases.

Gross Pathology Calcification of intervertebral disks and longitudinal ligaments.

Micro Pathology Similar to rheumatoid arthritis, but in different location and no rheumatoid nodules.

Treatment Physical therapy; nonsteroidal anti-inflammatory drugs (NSAIDs); sulfasalazine.

Discussion Also called Marie–Strümpell disease; associated with **HLA-B27;** this inflammatory arthritis with eventual ankylosis of the spine is typically seen in young males; longstanding cases may present with **iritis** and **aortic insufficiency;** also associated with Reiter's syndrome and inflammatory bowel disease.

ID/CC A 52-year-old white **female** complains to her family doctor of **difficulty climbing** steps for the past six months and difficulty washing her hair for the past two weeks.

HPI She states that she does not feel tired or short of breath but that her legs and arms "just will not cooperate." She also complains of intermittent fever.

PE **Periorbital edema** with purplish discoloration (= HELIOTROPE RASH); **butterfly rash** on face and neck; Raynaud's phenomenon; **scaling of skin with redness around knuckles** (= GOTTRON'S LESIONS); **proximal muscle weakness with tenderness** in all four extremities.

Labs **Elevated serum creatine kinase (CK)**; elevated aldolase; elevated erythrocyte sedimentation rate (ESR); mild leukocytosis; **antinuclear antibodies (ANAs)** present, particularly against tRNA. EMG: spontaneous fibrillation.

Imaging N/A

Gross Pathology Muscle edema progressing to muscle atrophy and fibrosis.

Micro Pathology Lymphocytic infiltration, primarily in a perivascular fashion but also between muscle fibers on muscle biopsy; atrophy; fibrosis.

Treatment Corticosteroids; methotrexate; azathioprine (= IMURAN).

Discussion Idiopathic disorder primarily affecting older females; frequently associated with malignancy (e.g., ovarian carcinoma).

ID/CC	A 45-year-old woman visits an orthopedist because of an **inability to extend her fourth and fifth fingers.**
HPI	She has a longstanding history of **alcohol abuse** and has been to the emergency room several times for alcoholic gastritis.
PE	Mild icterus; palmar erythema; muscle wasting; malnourishment; abdomen reveals 2+ ascitic fluid (due to alcoholic liver damage); **fourth and fifth fingers of right hand reveal flexion contracture** with nodular thickening and thick bands of tissue palpable upon drawing examining finger across palm.
Labs	N/A
Imaging	N/A
Gross Pathology	Infiltration of palmar fascia with fibrous tissue and subsequent contraction deformity.
Micro Pathology	Infiltration of pretendinous fascia with myofibroblasts with fibrosis of pretendinous bands.
Treatment	Surgery (release of contractures and adhesions); frequently recurs.
Discussion	Also called palmar fibromatosis; of unknown etiology; associated with alcoholism and **manual labor**. Dupuytren's contracture associated with diabetes, alcoholism, and anticonvulsant medications.

Hand–Schüller–Christian Disease

ID/CC	A 2-year-old boy is brought in for a pediatric consultation because his parents are concerned about **the child's protruding eyes** (= EXOPHTHALMOS) and **excessive urine volume** (= POLYURIA).
HPI	The parents also state that the child has been febrile and has had multiple ear infections.
PE	Low weight for age; bilateral exophthalmos; **painful swellings over head** (due to cystic bony lesions); no icterus; no lymphadenopathy; mild hepatosplenomegaly.
Labs	CBC: normal blood counts. **Increased serum osmolality**; **decreased urine osmolality**.
Imaging	XR-Skull: **multiple rounded lytic lesions.**
Gross Pathology	N/A
Micro Pathology	Granulomatous lesions and characteristic Langerhans cells with coffee-bean-shaped nuclei and pale, abundant cytoplasm on bone biopsy from skull lesions; **tennis-racket-shaped tubular structures** (= BIRBECK GRANULES) on electron microscopy; positive S-100 protein and CD1 antigen.
Treatment	Combination chemotherapy, curettage of bony lesions.
Discussion	A type of **Langerhans cell histiocytosis;** Hand–Schüller–Christian syndrome is multifocal, producing **diabetes insipidus** due to involvement of hypothalamus and exophthalmos from orbital infiltration by histiocytes.

ID/CC A 10-year-old male presents with a persistent **low-grade fever, skin rash, and painful swelling of both knees.**

HPI He also complains of excessive fatigue and significant anorexia. He has no history of sore throat, pedal edema/orthopnea, nocturnal dyspnea, or involuntary movements.

PE VS: fever. PE: extensive erythematous maculopapular rash; generalized lymphadenopathy; hepatosplenomegaly; arthritis of both knees; no subcutaneous nodules; no evidence of carditis; no Roth's spots on funduscopy; no petechiae over skin or mucosa; normal cardiovascular exam.

Labs CBC/PBS: leukocytosis; normocytic, normochromic anemia. Elevated erythrocyte sedimentation rate (ESR); blood cultures sterile; antistreptolysin O (ASO) titers normal; throat swab sterile; **rheumatoid factor negative;** leukocytosis with **elevated proteins and markedly low glucose and complement levels** on synovial fluid analysis. ECG: normal.

Imaging XR-Knees: effusion and soft tissue swelling. Echo: no vegetations or valvular disease.

Gross Pathology N/A

Micro Pathology N/A

Treatment Nonsteroidal anti-inflammatory drugs (NSAIDs); corticosteroids.

Discussion Juvenile rheumatoid arthritis (JRA) most commonly affects the knee joint. Patients with JRA should undergo periodic ophthalmologic exams to carefully monitor for onset of **iridocyclitis,** which can lead to blindness.

Mixed Connective Tissue Disorder (MCTD)

ID/CC A 42-year-old woman presents with **dysphagia, butterfly rash,** arthralgias, myalgias, **skin stiffness,** swelling of the fingers, **proximal muscle weakness,** and **chronic pain in the finger joints.**

HPI She has had these symptoms intermittently over the years, but they have worsened over the past year.

PE VS: normotension. PE: erythematous rash over face in butterfly distribution; **sclerodactyly;** telangiectasias in periungual areas; **nonerosive arthritis of wrist and ankle joints; proximal muscle weakness** and tenderness; weakness of neck muscles; no sensory loss; normal tendon reflexes; positive **Raynaud's phenomenon.**

Labs Elevated erythrocyte sedimentation rate (ESR); diffuse hypergammaglobulinemia; positive rheumatoid factor; high titer of antinuclear antibodies (speckled pattern); **strongly positive test for antibody to RNP antigen** (most typical finding); anti-Smith antibody negative; anti-dsDNA antibody negative; normal complement levels; elevated **serum creatine phosphokinase (CPK)** levels; muscle biopsy and EMG suggestive of polymyositis; **normal renal function tests.**

Imaging N/A

Gross Pathology N/A

Micro Pathology N/A

Treatment Corticosteroids and nonsteroidal anti-inflammatory drugs (NSAIDs).

Discussion MCTD includes characteristics of **one or more traditional connective tissue diseases at same time,** thus making it hard to label as one or the other. These disorders include systemic lupus erythematosus, scleroderma, rheumatoid arthritis, and polymyositis.

ID/CC   An obese 16-year-old male goes to a clinic because of **distal muscle weakness** in both upper and lower limbs and **gradual diminution of vision.**

HPI   His **father** suffered from a **similar muscular weakness.** The patient also suffers from mental retardation.

PE   **Frontal balding;** typical **facial wasting;** bilateral cataracts; **distal muscle weakness** in both upper and lower limbs; difficulty releasing grip after handshake; **percussion over tongue and thenar eminence reveals myotonia;** mildly reduced deep tendon reflexes; normal sensory exam; moderately **atrophic testicles;** equinovarus deformity of both feet.

Labs   **Decreased plasma IgG.** EMG: myopathic potentials; myotonia.

Imaging   ECG: Nonspecific ST-T changes.

Gross Pathology   N/A

Micro Pathology   Muscle biopsy reveals internal nuclei (nuclei in center of the fiber rather than in periphery), type I fiber atrophy, and ring fibers.

Treatment   Phenytoin; carbamazepine; quinidine; procainamide; acetazolamide; surgery required to correct foot deformities.

Discussion   Most common form of muscular dystrophy among **whites;** transmitted as **autosomal-dominant** trait. Genetic defect that encodes **myotonin protein kinase;** myotonic dystrophy gene locus has been mapped at chromosome 19q13.3.

Paget's Disease of Bone

ID/CC A 70-year-old male immigrant from England presents with **pain** in the right leg, producing an awkward gait, together with bilateral **hearing loss.**

HPI He has also noted a progressive **increase in his hat size.**

PE Slight **bowing of right tibia;** normal rectal exam; mixed conductive and **sensorineural hearing loss** confirmed by audiometry; physical exam otherwise normal.

Labs **Markedly elevated alkaline phosphatase;** mildly elevated serum calcium and phosphorus; normal serum transaminases; **increased urinary excretion of hydroxyproline.**

Imaging XR-Skull: scattered **islands of bone lysis** (= OSTEOPOROSIS CIRCUMSCRIPTA); mixed **thickening** (blastic) **and lucency** (lytic) of bone (= COTTON-WOOL APPEARANCE). XR-Leg (right side): bone soft with disorganized trabecular pattern; bowed tibia.

Gross Pathology Expansion of bone cortex, blastic bone lesions, and bowing of long bones (thick ivory bones).

Micro Pathology Multiple cement lines with unmineralized osteoid; indicative of excessive osteoblastic and osteoclastic activity.

Treatment Osteotomies; calcitonin; diphosphonate; mithramycin.

Discussion Disease of probable viral etiology; characterized by osteoclastic destruction of bone initially with excessive osteoblastic repair, producing bone sclerosis. When extensive, resulting increased blood flow leads to **high cardiac output congestive heart failure.** Other complications are **pathologic fracture and osteosarcoma** (1% of patients).

ID/CC A 44-year-old **male** with a history of hypertension develops sudden abdominal pain (due to mesenteric thrombosis) far more severe than prior episodes.

HPI The patient had a previous episode of hematuria with peripheral edema that was diagnosed as glomerulonephritis. He has a history of intermittent fever, malaise, myalgia, arthralgia, and other vague systemic symptoms.

PE **Livedo reticularis;** subcutaneous nodules of forearms and finger pads; painful, tympanic abdomen; purpuric spots in lower legs; **radial and peroneal nerve involvement** (= MONONEURITIS MULTIPLEX).

Labs CBC: marked neutrophilic **leukocytosis** with eosinophilia. Elevated erythrocyte sedimentation rate (ESR); **presence of hepatitis B surface antigen (HBSAg); positive P-ANCA.**

Imaging Angio-Renal: **multiple small aneurysms** and infarcts.

Gross Pathology Fibrinoid necrotizing inflammatory infiltrate of media and adventitia of small and medium-size vessels in segmental fashion, with thrombosis and possible aneurysm formation.

Micro Pathology Segmental areas of fibrinoid necrosis with neutrophilic infiltration of arterial wall.

Treatment Steroids and other immunosuppressive agents.

Discussion **Type III hypersensitivity reaction** characterized by **multisystem** involvement. **Renal involvement** most common, but other presentations include pericarditis, myocardial infarction, retinal occlusion, and asthma.

ID/CC A 37-year-old white female complains of **increasing weakness** for several months, especially on climbing stairs and while combing her hair.

HPI She also complains of **difficulty holding her neck upright.** For the past few weeks, she has also had **difficulty swallowing.**

PE Atrophy of neck, shoulder, and thigh muscles; motor weakness in all proximal muscle groups; no sensory deficit; deep tendon reflexes reduced; heliotrope and Gottron's papules seen in addition to photosensitive rash in exposed areas.

Labs Markedly elevated serum creatine phosphokinase (CPK) levels; antinuclear antibodies (ANAs) demonstrable; elevated serum transaminases and aldolase. EMG: markedly increased insertional activity; polyphasic low-amplitude motor unit action potentials with abnormally low recruitment.

Imaging N/A

Gross Pathology Muscle edema progressing to muscle atrophy and fibrosis.

Micro Pathology Biopsy from thigh muscles reveals **inflammatory infiltrate** in muscle, destruction of muscle fibers, and perivascular infiltrate of mononuclear cells; residual muscle fibers small.

Treatment High-dose glucocorticoids; methotrexate; azathioprine.

Discussion Frequently seen as **paraneoplastic** manifestation of ovarian, breast, uterine, or intestinal malignancy. An associated neoplasm should always be sought.

ID/CC   A 40-year-old white female complains of **paleness and bluish discoloration of the hands, mainly upon exposure to cold, with redness upon rewarming** (= RAYNAUD'S PHENOMENON), together with increasing pain in the knees, elbows, and hands over several months and recent **difficulty swallowing** solid food.

HPI   She also has **mask-like facies** with a limited range of expression.

PE   **Smooth, shiny, tight skin** over face and fingers; edema of hands and feet; palpable subcutaneous **calcinosis; pigmentation** and telangiectasias of face.

Labs   CBC: anemia. Hypergammaglobulinemia; anti-SCL-70 antibody; positive rheumatoid factor. PFTs: restrictive lung disease (fibrosis).

Imaging   UGI: loss of esophageal motility; dilated esophagus.

Gross Pathology   Pulmonary fibrosis with "honeycomb" appearance; swelling of esophageal wall; malabsorption syndrome; enlarged kidneys with areas of infarction; myocarditis and pericarditis.

Micro Pathology   Dense fibrosis of collagen tissue of dermis with loss of appendages and epidermal atrophy; intimal thickening of blood vessels, primarily in kidney but also in gastrointestinal tract and heart.

Treatment   Supportive; calcium channel blockers; omeprazole; cisapride; penicillamine.

Discussion   May be localized or systemic (visceral involvement); may present with calcinosis, Raynaud's phenomenon, esophageal involvement, sclerodactyly, and telangiectasia (= CREST SYNDROME).

ID/CC	A 23-year-old man presents with bilateral **conjunctivitis**, painful **swelling of the right knee,** bilateral heel pain, and **painless ulcers on his penis.**
HPI	He was diagnosed and treated for nongonococcal urethritis one week ago.
PE	Bilateral conjunctivitis with anterior uveitis; **circinate balanitis; kerato-blennorrhagicum on palms and soles;** arthritis of right knee and ankle.
Labs	**HLA-B27 positive;** synovial fluid reveals monocytes with phagocytosed neutrophils (= REITER CELLS); rheumatoid factor negative; elevated erythrocyte sedimentation rate (ESR).
Imaging	XR-Right Knee and Ankle: presence of **joint effusion.**
Gross Pathology	N/A
Micro Pathology	N/A
Treatment	Nonsteroidal anti-inflammatory drugs (NSAIDs) are mainstay of therapy; treat chlamydial urethritis with doxycycline.
Discussion	Reiter's syndrome is an HLA-B27-associated seronegative spondyloarthropathy that is seen almost exclusively in males and is associated with conjunctivitis, urethritis, arthritis, and heel pain. Condition has traditionally been classified as a sexually transmitted disease, but it has also occurred following regional enteritis with *Salmonella, Shigella, Campylobacter,* and *Yersinia.*

ID/CC   A 47-year-old white **female** visits her family doctor complaining of painful swelling of the right knee.

HPI   She has a history of chronic pain along with **morning stiffness** in the hand joints **lasting** for at least **two hours.**

PE   **Symmetrical deforming arthropathy** (ulnar deviation); soft-tissue swelling and tenderness in proximal interphalangeal and metacarpophalangeal (MCP) joint; wasting of small muscles of hand; flexion of MCP joint; extension of proximal interphalangeal (PIP) joint and flexion of distal interphalangeal (DIP) joint (= SWAN-NECK DEFORMITY); effusion on right knee with overlying skin redness and increased temperature; subcutaneous nodules.

Labs   Increased erythrocyte sedimentation rate (ESR); increased protein and white count in the synovial fluid; **positive rheumatoid factor** (IgM or IgA against IgG); positive antinuclear antibodies (ANAs); polyclonal gammopathy; associated with HLA-DR4.

Imaging   XR-Plain: narrowing of joint spaces; fusion of joint (= ANKYLOSIS); demineralization and bone erosions; juxta-articular osteoporosis.

Gross Pathology   Bone erosion with ankylosis; pericarditis, pleuritis; subcutaneous nodules with granuloma formation.

Micro Pathology   Plasma cell infiltration of synovial membranes (= SYNOVITIS) with destruction of articular cartilage, tendons, and ligaments by thickened, **inflamed synovial tissue** (= PANNUS); fibrosis.

Treatment   Physical therapy, thermal compresses, splints; nonsteroidal anti-inflammatory drugs (NSAIDs); methotrexate; gold; chloroquine; corticosteroids; other immunosuppressants; surgery.

Discussion   Most **common autoimmune disease;** ocular involvement seen in 5% of cases; neurologic involvement of carpal tunnel can be complication.

ID/CC   A 47-year-old woman visits her health care center complaining of **dryness of the mouth** (= XEROSTOMIA) and a **gritty sensation in her eyes with dryness** (= XEROPHTHALMIA).

HPI   She has been hypertensive for 20 years and has suffered from longstanding **rheumatoid arthritis,** for which she has been treated with nonsteroidal anti-inflammatory drugs (NSAIDs).

PE   **Filamentous keratitis with areas of denuded corneal epithelium** (= KERATOCONJUNCTIVITIS SICCA) on slit-lamp examination with rose bengal dye staining of cornea; **diminished tear formation** as measured on strip of filter paper, with one end of paper placed inside lower eyelid (= SCHIRMER TEST); **parotid enlargement;** excessively dry mouth with abundant dental caries; characteristic swan-neck deformities of hands and ulnar deviation (due to longstanding deforming rheumatoid arthritis).

Labs   Low saliva flow rates with lemon juice stimulation (< 0.5 ml/min); hypergammaglobulinemia; **positive antibodies to IgG globulins** (= RHEUMATOID FACTOR) and **antinuclear antibodies (ANAs).**

Imaging   Sialography (x-rays following cannulation and contrast injection of parotid ducts): distortion of normal arborization pattern. Nuc: impaired salivary function.

Gross Pathology   N/A

Micro Pathology   Salivary and lacrimal glands show inflammatory infiltration with T cells, B cells, and plasma cells, with predominance of CD4+ T cells; **ductal obstruction** with glandular acinar tissue atrophy with fatty change.

Treatment   Artificial tear preparations, increased and frequent oral intake of fluids, careful dental hygiene, plaque control programs, fluoride application.

Discussion   Autoimmune destruction of salivary and lacrimal glands; may be primary or associated with other autoimmune diseases.

Systemic Lupus Erythematosus (SLE)

ID/CC An 18-year-old white **female** presents with a **malar rash** that is exacerbated by sun exposure (= PHOTOSENSITIVITY) as well as with arthralgias, and **joint stiffness** involving her ankles, wrists, and knee joints; she also complains of decreased visual acuity, anorexia, weight loss, malaise, and weakness.

HPI She has a history of hematuria and no history of drug intake prior to the onset of symptoms.

PE VS: hypertension (BP 160/100). PE: pallor; malar rash; painful restriction of movement of wrist, knee, and ankle joints; no obvious deformity; whitish exudates in cytoid bodies on funduscopic exam.

Labs CBC: Coombs-positive **anemia; neutropenia; thrombocytopenia. Decreased C3, C4; positive antinuclear antibodies (ANAs), anti-native DNA, and anti-Sm antibodies;** positive LE cells; false-positive VDRL due to anti-phospholipid antibodies. UA: proteinuria; red blood cells (RBCs) and **RBC casts.**

Imaging XR-Plain: no erosive changes. Echo: no vegetations seen on valves (vs. endocarditis).

Gross Pathology Serositis; pericarditis; pleuritis; splenomegaly; hyperkeratotic, erythematous plaques.

Micro Pathology Thickening of basement membrane on renal biopsy; mesangial proliferation; thickened capillary walls, creating **"wire-loop"** appearance; diffuse proliferative glomerulonephritis; immune complex deposition in skin with lymphocytic infiltration; vasculitis with fibrinoid necrosis of small arteries; almost any organ may be involved.

Treatment High-dose corticosteroids for prolonged periods; alternative drugs: chloroquine; cyclophosphamide as treatment for lupus nephritis.

Discussion **Type III hypersensitivity reaction;** immune complex vasculitis is basic pathologic lesion; can be drug-induced (e.g., hydralazine, procainamide, isoniazid).

Acute Tubular Necrosis (ATN)

ID/CC
A 17-year-old white male undergoing chemotherapy for disseminated Hodgkin's lymphoma complains of severe headaches, nausea, and weight loss.

HPI
The patient had been on **aminoglycosides.** When questioned, he is uncertain of place and time, but despite his confusion he describes his urine as appearing reddish-orange over the past few weeks.

PE
Confused but alert; underweight; no acute distress.

Labs
Lytes: increased potassium. UA: **oliguria;** hematuria; mild proteinuria; granular casts in urine; renal tubular epithelial cells in sediment; isotonic urine osmolality; **elevated urinary sodium** (> 40 mEq/L). Increased serum inorganic phosphorus; **azotemia** with blood urea nitrogen (BUN)/creatinine ratio of five (within normal limits).

Imaging
N/A

Gross Pathology
Kidneys enlarged, flabby, and pale with edema.

Micro Pathology
Necrosis of tubular epithelial cells that slough into lumen, forming casts and causing blockade; hydropic degeneration of epithelium.

Treatment
Discontinue offending agent; fluid and electrolyte management.

Discussion
Acute tubular damage resulting in acute renal failure; caused by prolonged ischemia or toxins (nephrotoxic drugs).

Adult Polycystic Kidney Disease (APKD)

ID/CC   A 47-year-old white male enters the emergency room complaining of a sudden-onset, **severe headache** that is the **"worst headache of his life."**

HPI   He also describes slow-onset dull pain in his left flank together with blood in his urine. He was recently treated for **recurrent urinary tract infections,** which were attributed to an enlarged prostate gland. His **father** died of **chronic renal failure,** and his paternal **grandfather** died of **cerebral hemorrhage.**

PE   VS: hypertension (BP 170/110). PE: palpable, nontender **abdominal mass** on both flanks; nuchal rigidity.

Labs   UA: albuminuria; microscopic **hematuria** (no white blood cells or casts). Slightly increased blood urea nitrogen (BUN), creatinine.

Imaging   Angio-Neuro: ruptured **berry aneurysm.** CT/US-Abdomen: **multiple kidney and liver cysts.**

Gross Pathology   Kidneys markedly enlarged and heavy with hundreds of cysts that almost replace normal parenchyma; cysts thick-walled, ranging from a few millimeters to several centimeters in diameter.

Micro Pathology   Cystic dilatation of tubules; epithelial cell hyperplasia; cuboidal epithelium lining cysts.

Treatment   Dialysis and renal transplantation.

Discussion   Autosomal-dominant disease caused by defect in **chromosome 16** in which renal parenchyma converted to hundreds of fluid-filled cysts, resulting in progressive renal failure in adulthood. Cysts may also involve pancreas, liver, lungs, and spleen; associated with berry aneurysms of circle of Willis, hypertension, and mitral valve prolapse.

ID/CC	A 5-year-old **female** is brought to the pediatrician because her mother noticed **blood in her urine** and **diminished vision acuity.**
HPI	Her family is **Mormon.** Her mother suffers from chronic renal failure.
PE	VS: normotension. PE: appears well nourished; bilateral **sensorineural hearing loss;** bilateral **cataracts.**
Labs	CBC/PBS: normochromic, normocytic **anemia.** High-tone sensorineural loss detected on audiometry; elevated serum creatinine and blood urea nitrogen (BUN). UA: **proteinuria; hematuria;** red blood cell (RBC) casts.
Imaging	N/A
Gross Pathology	Small, smooth kidneys.
Micro Pathology	Longitudinal thinning and splitting of glomerular basement membrane, producing characteristic laminated appearance with glomerular sclerosis; interstitial infiltrate containing fat-filled macrophages (= LARGE FOAM CELLS).
Treatment	Angiotensin-converting enzyme (ACE) inhibitors; renal transplantation.
Discussion	Probably autosomal-dominant; caused by defect in alpha chain of type IV collagen. Also called hereditary chronic nephritis. Progressive in males.

ID/CC A 56-year-old male complains of **urinary frequency** and interruption of the urinary stream over the past six months; he also complains of having to wake up multiple times during the night to urinate (= NOCTURIA).

HPI The patient's history includes one episode of acute urinary retention one month ago that was relieved with catheterization. He denies any history of hematuria (vs. carcinoma of the bladder) or back pain (vs. metastasized prostatic carcinoma). He also admits to having a **reduced caliber of urine stream** and **terminal dribbling** as well as **urinary hesitancy.**

PE **Smooth enlargement of the prostate** protruding into the rectum on digital rectal exam; overlying rectal mucosa mobile; **bladder percussible up to umbilicus.**

Labs UA: 2+ bacteria; positive nitrite and leukocyte esterase. Prostate-specific antigen (PSA) levels normal; urodynamic studies demonstrate **bladder neck obstruction** with increased residual urine volume; mildly elevated serum creatinine and blood urea nitrogen (BUN).

Imaging US: benign-appearing enlargement of median lobe.

Gross Pathology Enlarged prostate with well-demarcated nodules up to 1 cm in diameter in **median lobe** of prostate.

Micro Pathology Both stroma and glands show hyperplasia; fibromyoadenomatous hyperplasia seen in which proliferating glands are surrounded by proliferating smooth muscle cells and fibroblasts.

Treatment Finasteride; transurethral resection of prostate (TURP). Treat associated urinary tract infections with appropriate antibiotics (e.g., SMX-TMP, ciprofloxacin).

Discussion Age-dependent changes of estrogens and androgens are believed to cause BPH; increasing incidence noted starting at 40 years of age; affects up to 75% of men by age of 80 years.

ID/CC A 48-year-old white female is admitted to the hospital because of worsening **generalized edema** and weakness along with **hypertension.**

HPI She has a long history of **insulin-dependent diabetes mellitus (IDDM)** but no history of hematuria, recent sore throat, or skin infections.

PE VS: **hypertension** (BP 160/110). PE: **generalized pitting edema;** no evidence of pleural effusion or ascites; lung bases clear on auscultation; jugular venous pressure normal; neither kidney palpable; funduscopic exam reveals presence of **proliferative diabetic retinopathy.**

Labs **Elevated** fasting **blood sugar** (234 mg/dL); elevated glycosylated hemoglobin (10%); **elevated blood urea nitrogen (BUN) and serum creatinine; decreased serum albumin; elevated blood cholesterol.** UA: presence of sugar and **3+ protein;** broad casts and **fatty casts;** elevated quantitative protein (3.5 gm/24 hr).

Imaging N/A

Gross Pathology N/A

Micro Pathology Increased mesangial matrix on renal biopsy; thickening of capillary basement membrane combined with acellular eosinophilic nodules in mesangium (= KIMMELSTIEL–WILSON DISEASE); hyaline arteriosclerosis of both afferent and efferent arterioles; no immune complex deposits seen.

Treatment Blood sugar control; control of systemic hypertension, preferably with angiotensin-converting enzyme (ACE) inhibitor; dietary protein and phosphate restriction; avoidance of nephrotoxic drugs; dialysis or renal transplantation.

Discussion Diabetic glomerulosclerosis is renal manifestation of diabetic microangiopathy; presents at least 10 years after diabetes appears (more commonly in IDDM); usually prelude to end-stage diabetic renal disease.

IgA Nephropathy (Berger's Disease)

ID/CC	A 22-year-old white male complains of recurrent episodes of **"bloody urine"** that lasted for several days **in conjunction** with an **upper respiratory tract infection.**
HPI	He was well until the onset of symptoms.
PE	Pallor; slight palpebral edema; remainder of PE within normal limits.
Labs	UA: proteinuria; **red cell casts in urine;** gross hematuria. **Increased serum IgA.**
Imaging	N/A
Gross Pathology	N/A
Micro Pathology	Focal glomerulonephritis involving only selected glomeruli with mesangial proliferation and segmental necrosis with crescents; IgA deposits with some IgM, IgG, and C3 on immunofluorescence.
Treatment	Supportive.
Discussion	Idiopathic but associated with upper respiratory or gastrointestinal infections lacking latency period (vs. poststreptococcal glomerulonephritis). The glomerular pathology seen in Berger's disease is similar to that seen in **Henoch–Schönlein purpura,** which is seen in children. **Chronic renal failure may ultimately develop.**

ID/CC   An 11-year-old white girl is brought to the pediatrician because of headache, chest palpitations, and ringing in her ears together with **generalized edema.**

HPI   She has no history of dyspnea, sore throat, skin infections, or fever. Careful questioning reveals that she has also had **hematuria.**

PE   VS: hypertension (BP 140/100). PE: **generalized** (including periorbital) **pitting edema;** jugular venous pressure normal; lung bases clear; neither kidney palpable; no evidence of pleural effusion or ascites.

Labs   Elevated blood urea nitrogen (BUN) and serum creatinine; decreased serum albumin; elevated serum triglycerides; serum **hypocomplementemia;** antinuclear antibody (ANA) negative; normal antistreptolysin-O (ASO) titers. UA: **fatty casts and oval bodies in addition to proteins.**

Imaging   N/A

Gross Pathology   N/A

Micro Pathology   Diffuse glomerular involvement with thickened capillary walls and lobular mesangial proliferation on light microscopy. Splitting of basement membrane causing **railroad-track appearance** with periodic acid-Schiff (PAS) reagent or silver stain; **prominent granular immunofluorescence;** mesangial and subendothelial deposits of immune complexes.

Treatment   Corticosteroids; renal transplantation.

Discussion   Idiopathic; may be associated inherited deficiencies of complement components and partial lipodystrophy. Subdivided into two types: type I MPGN (both classic and alternative complement pathways activated) and type II MPGN (dense deposit disease; activation of alternate complement pathway). Approximately 50% of patients with MPGN will go on to develop **chronic renal failure.** There is a **high recurrence rate** post renal transplantation.

ID/CC   A 64-year-old man is admitted to the internal medicine ward because of **generalized edema** (= ANASARCA).

HPI   Six months ago, the patient was diagnosed with **lung cancer.** He has smoked three packs of cigarettes per day for 20 years. He has no history of dyspnea, throat or skin infections, fever, hematuria, hypertension, or diabetes.

PE   VS:**hypertension** (BP 150/100). PE: **generalized pitting edema;** no evidence of pleural effusion or ascites; jugular venous pressure normal; lung bases clear; neither kidney palpable; no hepatosplenomegaly.

Labs   CBC: normal. **Hypoalbuminemia; increased serum cholesterol;** mildly elevated blood urea nitrogen (BUN) and serum creatinine; mildly reduced complement levels, hepatitis B surface antigen (HBsAg) negative. UA: **massive proteinuria; fatty casts and oval fat bodies.**

Imaging   N/A

Gross Pathology   N/A

Micro Pathology   Diffuse thickening of glomerular basement membrane and capillary wall with little increase in cellularity; subepithelial deposits between glomerular basement membrane and epithelial cells on electron microscopy; diffuse capillary wall deposition of IgG and C3 in **granular or lumpy-bumpy pattern** on **immunofluorescence** secondary to circulating immune complex deposition.

Treatment   Corticosteroids, cyclophosphamide, dialysis, renal transplantation.

Discussion   Most **common cause of nephrotic syndrome** in adults; may be idiopathic or secondary to drugs (penicillamine, captopril), connective tissue diseases, or malignancy.

Minimal Change Disease

ID/CC   A **5-year-old** white male presents with **generalized edema** and abdominal distention, producing respiratory embarrassment.

HPI   The child had an **upper respiratory infection** one week ago.

PE   VS: normotension. PE: generalized pitting edema; free **ascitic fluid** in peritoneal cavity; shifting dullness and fluid thrill present; normal funduscopic exam.

Labs   UA: 4+ **proteinuria** (more than 3 g/24 hrs). **Hypoalbuminemia; hypercholesterolemia;** hypertriglyceridemia; decreased serum ionic calcium; normal C3 levels; moderately elevated serum creatinine and blood urea nitrogen (BUN).

Imaging   N/A

Gross Pathology   Kidneys slightly enlarged, soft, and yellowish.

Micro Pathology   Light microscopy and immunofluorescent studies **normal on renal biopsy** (no evidence of immune complex deposition).

Treatment   Corticosteroids; salt-restricted diet; diuretics; electrolyte therapy and monitoring.

Discussion   Also called **lipoid nephrosis;** most common cause of idiopathic nephrotic syndrome in children; associated with infections or vaccinations. **Good prognosis.**

ID/CC   A 47-year-old black diabetic female complains of weight loss, progressive shortness of breath, and **swelling of the lower legs** and arms.

HPI   Her past medical history is unremarkable.

PE   Pallor; pitting edema in extremities; decreased lung sounds with crackles bilaterally in lower lung fields; **periorbital edema; ascites.**

Labs   UA: **proteinuria** (> 3.5 g/24 hr); lipiduria with oval fat bodies and fatty and waxy casts in urinary sediment. **Hypoalbuminemia** (< 3 g/dL); **hyperlipidemia** (serum cholesterol 250 mg/dL).

Imaging   N/A

Gross Pathology   Kidneys enlarged, pale, and rubbery; renal vein thrombosis may be present.

Micro Pathology   Thickened basement membrane; deposits of IgG and C3 along basement membrane seen in **"spike and dome"** pattern on methenamine silver stain; immune deposits in a **"lumpy-bumpy"** (discontinuous) pattern on immunofluorescence.

Treatment   Corticosteroids; cyclophosphamide; renal transplantation; acetylcholinesterase (ACE) inhibitors reduce urinary protein loss.

Discussion   May be idiopathic or caused by membranous glomerulonephritis (most common cause in adults), minimal change disease (= LIPOID NEPHROSIS) (most common in children), focal glomerulosclerosis, or membranoproliferative glomerulonephritis. Patients with nephrotic syndrome have **hypercoagulability** secondary to loss of antithrombin III in the urine (e.g., increased incidence of peripheral vein thrombosis).

ID/CC A 56-year-old **male Thai immigrant** complains of **painless hematuria** of several days' duration.

HPI He is a **heavy smoker** and once loved to swim in a **lake** in his hometown that was known to harbor many **snails** (risk of schistosomiasis transmission).

PE Lungs clear: abdomen nontender; no palpable masses; genitalia within normal limits; no lymphadenopathy.

Labs CBC: slight normocytic, normochromic anemia. UA: **hematuria** and abundant epithelial cells. Remainder of routine blood work and stool studies normal.

Imaging IVP/Cystogram: **irregular filling defects** above trigone.

Gross Pathology Nodular, cauliflower-like lesion with central necrosis and minimal invasion of bladder wall.

Micro Pathology Cytology of urine shows malignant cells. Biopsy of bladder shows grade I, stage B **transitional cell carcinoma** (TCC) arising from uroepithelium and projecting into bladder.

Treatment Surgery (aggressive fulguration); radiotherapy; chemotherapy.

Discussion Fourfold increase in risk in men. Risk factors include industrial exposure to **arylamines, cigarette smoke,** *Schistosoma haematobium* infection, **analgesic abuse** (especially phenacetin), and **cyclophosphamide** therapy. Complications include invasion of perivesicular tissue, ureteral invasion with urinary obstruction (leading to hydronephrosis, pyelonephritis, and renal failure), and metastases to lung, bone, and liver. Transitional cell carcinoma appears to be associated with mutations in the p53 tumor suppressor gene and deletions in chromosome 9q.

ID/CC   A 45-year-old white female complains of palpitations and shortness of breath; morning swelling of the eyes, arms, and legs; and numbness of the lower legs.

HPI   Her past medical history is unremarkable.

PE   VS: **cardiac arrhythmia** on auscultation. PE: mild cardiomegaly; **macroglossia;** pitting **edema** in lower extremities; **ascites**.

Labs   UA: proteinuria. ECG: ventricular hypertrophy and low voltage (restrictive cardiomyopathy). Hypoproteinemia; hyperlipidemia.

Imaging   CXR: biventricular cardiac enlargement.

Gross Pathology   Pathologic deposition of amyloid glycoprotein in several organs, primarily heart and kidney; kidneys pale, waxy, gray, and firm; spleen and liver may be enlarged; deep-brown discoloration characteristic of amyloid-infiltrated organs exposed to iodine.

Micro Pathology   **Apple-green birefringence** in polarized light when stained **with Congo red;** amyloid deposition in mesangium as well as in endothelium surrounding hepatic sinusoids and in spleen; hyaline thickening of arteriolar walls, leading to narrowing of lumen and ischemia.

Treatment   Supportive.

Discussion   Commonly presents with nephrotic syndrome; can be primary or secondary to B-cell dyscrasias such as those of multiple myeloma, chronic inflammatory states, and tuberculosis.

ID/CC　A 68-year-old **black** male complains of **dysuria, progressively increased urinary frequency,** and **back pain** that has lasted several months.

HPI　He reports **high animal-fat intake.**

PE　Nodular, **rock-hard, irregular area of induration** in **peripheral lobe** of prostate on digital rectal exam; **midline furrow** between prostatic lobes **obscured; extension to seminal vesicles** detected.

Labs　**Markedly elevated prostate-specific antigen (PSA)** and **acid phosphatase.**

Imaging　Transrectal US-Prostate: **Hypoechoic masses** in peripheral zone with extension to seminal vesicles. Nuc-Bone Scan: **hot lesions of spine, sacrum, and pelvic bones** (axial skeleton). CT/MR: prostate mass with capsular penetration and enlarged seminal vesicles.

Gross Pathology　Irregularly enlarged, firm, nodular prostate.

Micro Pathology　Core Needle Biopsy-Prostate: single layer of malignant neoplastic cells arranged haphazardly in adenoplastic stroma.

Treatment　Prostatectomy with radiation; orchiectomy; leuprolide; androgens; flutamide.

Discussion　Primary malignant neoplasm of prostate commonly arising from peripheral zone (70%). The **most common male cancer.** Prognosis and treatment depend heavily on stage. Prostate cancer exhibits **hematogenous dissemination,** most commonly to **bone,** forming **osteoblastic lesions.** Tumor can also invade sacral nerve roots, causing significant pain.

ID/CC   A 60-year-old white male complains of right **flank pain** and **hematuria.**

HPI   He has been a **heavy smoker** for the past 24 years; he **lost five pounds over the past month** and is not on a diet.

PE   VS: low-grade fever; moderate hypertension. PE: pallor; **palpable mass** in right flank.

Labs   **Elevated red blood cell mass** (= POLYCYTHEMIA); Elevated erythrocyte sedimentation rate (ESR). CBC/PBS: normocytic, normochromic **anemia.** UA: gross **hematuria.**

Imaging   IVP/CT/US: mass in upper pole of right kidney. MR: no invasion of renal vein or inferior vena cava (IVC).

Gross Pathology   Yellowish areas of necrotic tissue with focal areas of hemorrhage within renal parenchyma.

Micro Pathology   Clear cells (containing glycogen) with evidence of cytologic atypia invading renal parenchyma.

Treatment   Right nephrectomy; consider renal sparing partial nephrectomy.

Discussion   **Most common renal tumor.** Increased risk in **von Hippel–Lindau syndrome** and **acquired polycystic kidney disease.** Frequently invades renal vein and IVC. Metastasizes to lungs and bone via hematogenous dissemination; can cause **paraneoplastic syndromes** (erythropoietin, parathyroid hormone, adrenocorticotropic hormone [ACTH], and renin).

ID/CC	A 63-year-old white male complains of **sudden-onset pain in** the right **flank** together with gross **hematuria**, nausea, and vomiting.
HPI	He is **overweight,** has been diabetic for 15 years, is a heavy **smoker** and drinker, and has been surgically treated for **aortofemoral occlusive disease** (graft).
PE	VS: no fever; mild hypertension (BP 150/100). PE: **acute distress;** pallor; sweating; severe right flank pain; **xanthelasma** in both eyelids.
Labs	Normal blood urea nitrogen (BUN) and creatinine. UA: **hematuria**. ECG: old silent anterior wall myocardial infarction. Elevated **lactate dehydrogenase (LDH)**.
Imaging	CT-Abdomen: **wedge-shaped, nonenhancing lesion in right kidney**. US-Renal: edematous kidney with focal region of decreased color flow.
Gross Pathology	Wedge-shaped area of hemorrhagic necrosis in renal cortex.
Micro Pathology	Coagulation necrosis involving renal cortical nephrons extending into corticomedullary junction.
Treatment	Remove arterial obstruction by thrombolysis; heparin anticoagulation to prevent recurrence.
Discussion	Risk factors for embolic events include **atherosclerosis** and mural thrombi in heart and aorta, infectious endocarditis vegetations, and atheromatous plaques in aorta. Complications from renal artery embolism include renal failure, hypertension, acute pyelonephritis, and renal abscess.

Renal Stones (Nephrolithiasis)

ID/CC	A 35-year-old white male suddenly develops **severe,** colicky right **flank pain radiating to his right testicle,** as well as nausea and repeated vomiting.
HPI	He is admitted to the hospital for evaluation, at which time blood is drawn and a **urine** sample requested; the urine sample turns out to be **frankly bloody.**
PE	VS: mild tachycardia. PE: pallor; sweating; acute distress; **moving from one side of bed to the other;** right flank tenderness; right **costovertebral angle tenderness.**
Labs	UA: **hematuria;** abundant epithelial cells; some bacteria.
Imaging	KUB/IVP: radiopaque stone at right ureterovesicular junction. US: multiple small stones in right kidney.
Gross Pathology	N/A
Micro Pathology	N/A
Treatment	Pain relief; endoscopic removal of stone; high intake of fluids; open surgery (uretero-, pyelo-, or nephro-lithotomy); extracorporeal shock wave lithotripsy (ESWL).
Discussion	In the acute setting, patients with urinary stones typically present with **very severe pain** and cannot find a comfortable position in which to rest; **stones predispose to infection** and can lead to destruction of renal parenchyma. Most common type is calcium oxalate and phosphate; less common are magnesium ammonium phosphate, uric acid, and cystine. Approximately 85% of all renal stones are radiopaque; uric acid stones are radiolucent.

ID/CC	A 25-year-old white female develops **deep respirations** (= KUSSMAUL'S RESPIRATION), leg cramps, and muscle weakness.
HPI	She was diagnosed with Sjögren's syndrome two years ago and underwent kidney stone fragmentation (= LITHOTRIPSY) last year.
PE	Prominent **muscle weakness** with **hyporeflexia;** dryness of mouth (= XEROSTOMIA); dryness of eyes (= XEROPHTHALMIA); parotid enlargement.
Labs	Lytes: increased urinary potassium secretion with resulting **hypokalemia; hyperchloremic metabolic acidosis.** UA: alkaline urine; hypercalciuria. Decreased serum HCO_3; decreased serum inorganic phosphorus; normal calcium; high alkaline phosphatase.
Imaging	XR-Plain: osteomalacia, symmetric fractures of ribs and humeri. KUB: radiopaque genitourinary (GU) tract stones.
Gross Pathology	Complications can include nephrocalcinosis and osteomalacia.
Micro Pathology	N/A
Treatment	Bicarbonate; potassium; vitamin D.
Discussion	Metabolic acidosis caused by renal tubular defects in transport. Type I: selective deficiency of tubular H^+ secretion (hypokalemia); Type II: inability to reabsorb HCO_3 (hypokalemia); Type III: inability to produce NH_3 due to persistently low glomerular filtration rate (GFR) volumes (normokalemia); Type IV: primary or drug-induced hypoaldosteronism (hyperkalemia).

ID/CC A **36-year-old** male presents with **progressive painless enlargement of the left testicle** of two months' duration.

HPI He also complains of a sense of heaviness in his scrotum. He denies any history of pain or trauma at the site.

PE Walnut-sized, nontender, smooth, **firm mass at upper end of left testicle; mass does not transilluminate;** epididymis and vas deferens normal on palpation; prostate and seminal vesicles normal on digital rectal exam; abdominal lymph nodes not palpable; no hepatomegaly.

Labs Normal levels of human chorionic gonadotropin (hCG); **normal levels of serum alpha-fetoprotein and lactate dehydrogenase (LDH); histologic** diagnosis based on postoperative specimen study.

Imaging CXR: no metastasis. CT: no metastasis.

Gross Pathology Solid white bulging mass within testis.

Micro Pathology Sheets of germ cells with lymphocytes in fibrous stroma.

Treatment Orchiectomy with retroperitoneal lymph node dissection; chemotherapy with cisplatin; radiotherapy.

Discussion Dysgerminomas in ovaries are histologically similar. Tumors are extremely **radiosensitive.** Good prognosis; **cryptorchidism** predisposes to development of testicular tumors.

ID/CC	A 23-year-old white male is seen by his family physician because of **dyspnea, bilateral enlargement of the breasts** (= GYNECOMASTIA), and a **painless lump in the right testis** of approximately two months' duration.
HPI	He denies any history of sexually transmitted diseases, genital ulcers, drug use, or trauma.
PE	Bilateral nontender gynecomastia (due to increased human chorionic gonadotropin [hCG]); left supraclavicular lymphadenopathy; 5-cm **hard mass** palpable **on right testis,** distorting shape; normal rectal exam.
Labs	**Markedly elevated blood hCG and alpha-fetoprotein (AFP).**
Imaging	CXR: multiple bilateral **metastatic nodules** (= "CANNONBALL SECONDARIES"). US/MR-Testes: **solid intratesticular mass** with some foci of hemorrhage (intratesticular masses usually malignant).
Gross Pathology	N/A
Micro Pathology	Cytotrophoblastic and syncytiotrophoblastic cells with hCG demonstrable within cytoplasm.
Treatment	High radical inguinal orchiectomy followed by cisplatin-based combination chemotherapy.
Discussion	May be pure or mixed (mixed germ cell neoplasm); highly malignant with early and widespread metastasis. **Cryptorchidism** predisposes to development of testicular tumors.

ID/CC   A 9-year-old black male is brought into the emergency room because of **sudden-onset** severe **pain** that he experienced in the lower abdomen and **scrotum** while playing soccer.

HPI   He has no relevant medical history. Upon admission, he became nauseated and vomited three times.

PE   Irritability; right **testicle** tender, **swollen,** and elevated; palpable normal epididymis anteriorly; **increased pain with elevation of mass** (= PREHN'S SIGN); no hernia palpable; no transillumination of mass.

Labs   UA: mild leukocytosis.

Imaging   US-Scrotal: asymmetric decreased color flow in testicle. Nuc-Tc99: **doughnut sign** (due to central testicular ischemia and circumferential collateral flow).

Gross Pathology   Testicle markedly enlarged with hemorrhagic necrosis; scrotum may be purplish; cord twisted.

Micro Pathology   Severe venous congestion; interstitial hemorrhage; hemorrhagic necrosis.

Treatment   **Immediate surgery** due to risk of testicle loss (< 4 hours); contralateral orchiopexy prophylactically (high incidence of bilaterality); atrophic testicle should be removed due to possible autoimmune destruction of contralateral testis.

Discussion   Surgical emergency; needs to be differentiated from orchitis, epididymitis, and strangulated hernia. Seen more frequently in an **undescended testicle** (= CRYPTORCHIDISM).

ID/CC   A **3-year-old** male is brought to his pediatrician for evaluation of an **abdominal mass** that his parents noticed.

HPI   The child has been well all his life.

PE   Slight pallor; weight and height right for age; nontender, large, firm, and smooth intra-abdominal mass to right of midline; right **cryptorchidism** and **aniridia.**

Labs   UA: microscopic **hematuria;** urinary vanillylmandelic acid (VMA). Normal blood urea nitrogen (BUN); increased serum erythropoietin.

Imaging   IVP: displacement and distortion of right pelvicaliceal system. CT-Abdomen: tumor arising from right kidney with areas of low density (due to necrosis); persistent ellipsoid area of enhancement (due to compressed renal parenchyma); no evidence of vascular invasion.

Gross Pathology   Whitish, solid tumor with areas of hemorrhagic necrosis distorting normal renal parenchyma compressed into narrow rim; may be involvement of perirenal fat; metastasis usually to lungs.

Micro Pathology   Glomeruloid and tubular structures enclosed within spindle cell stroma; areas of cartilage, bone, or striated muscle tissue.

Treatment   Surgical removal of kidney containing tumor; chemotherapy with actinomycin and vincristine; radiotherapy.

Discussion   Malignant tumor of embryonal origin; associated with deletions on **chromosome 11** involving WT-1 gene; differentiated from neuroblastoma and malignant lymphoma, which are other small cell tumors of childhood. **WAGR syndrome** consists of Wilms' tumor, aniridia, genital abnormalities, and mental retardation. Also known as **nephroblastoma.**

About the Authors

VIKAS BHUSHAN, MD
Vikas is a diagnostic radiologist in Los Angeles and the series editor for *Underground Clinical Vignettes*. His interests include traveling, reading, writing, and world music. He is single and can be reached at vbhushan@aol.com.

CHIRAG AMIN, MD
Chirag is an orthopedics resident at Orlando Regional Medical Center. He can be reached at chiragamin@aol.com.

TAO LE, MD
Tao is completing a medicine residency at Yale-New Haven Hospital and is applying for a fellowship in allergy and immunology. He is married to Thao, who is a pediatrics resident. He can be reached at taotle@aol.com.

HOANG NGUYEN
Hoang (Henry) is a third-year MD/PhD student at Northwestern University. Henry is single and lives in Chicago, where he spends his free time writing, reading, and enjoying music. He can be reached at hbnguyen@nwu.edu.

JOSE M. FIERRO, MD
Jose (Pepe) is beginning a med/peds residency at Brookdale University Hospital in New York. He is a general surgeon from Mexico who worked extensively in Central Africa. His interests include world citizenship and ethnic music. He is married and can be reached at fierro@mail.dsinet.com.mx.

VISHAL PALL, MBBS
Vishal recently completed medical school and internship in Chandigarh, India. He hopes to begin his residency training in the US in July 1999. He can be reached at mona@puniv.chd.nic.in.

ALEXANDER GRIMM
Alexander (Alex) is a third-year medical student at the St. Louis University School of Medicine. His interests include computers. Alex is single and lives in St. Louis. He can be reached at grimma@slu.edu.